"There are so many myths, pre-conceptions, theories and varying approaches to street fighting, particularly when we have "traditional" martial artists professing to understand the complexities of street fighting and "real" combat, that this book makes a refreshing and enlightening change.

Kris, Lawrence and Erik, have masterfully demonstrated the key differences between training in these, sometimes, opposing arenas.

Having spent many years transitioning arts from the dojo to the street, I have to commend the authors on a job well done here. Protecting yourself and your loved ones isn't always as simple as using the most effective technique, there are far more variables and complexities that must be addressed, such as the environment, the level of threat or who the protagonist is (drunkle or attacker with murderous intent), and finally we have a manual that explains these in eloquent detail.

I've had the pleasure of training with Kris and Lawrence and their level of knowledge in all of the arts, combined with their ability to translate this to skills that can save your life, is quite simply, first class.

If you want an honest and effective instruction on how to handle confrontations that become a physical grapple, *Dirty Ground* has to be on the top of your list."

—**Al Peasland, author,** Self-Protection Instructor, Founder of Complete Self
Protection Ltd. (www.CompleteSelfProtection.com)

"At last! A book that addresses the reality that sport, fighting and self-defense are not "one size fits all" propositions.

This is a not just a practical reference for the serious martial art practitioner. It is an invaluable resource for martial art instructors who need to impress upon their students the "big picture" about the factors involved in self-defense situations in terms of reasonable levels of force and legal accountability.

The main premise of *Dirty Ground* is that different physical conflict scenarios are characterized by distinct factors requiring situation-specific considerations.

The book gives the martial artist or fighter the tools to understand and modify his or her own practice in preparation for a variety of possible types of encounters.

Dirty Ground is a highly readable, well organized, and clearly illustrated volume that should be on the shelf of any martial artist or fighter who is concerned about responsible self-defense and its consequences, both moral and legal."

—**Linda Yiannakis, M.S.,** 5th Dan Judo (USA Judo/ USJJF), 4th dan Jujutsu
(USJJF), Member, National Board of Advisors, Institute of Traditional Martial Arts at UNM

"Not only does *Dirty Ground* fill a void in the martial arts book genre, but it also fills a void in martial arts training. Wilder and Kane show us that critically important place that exists between sport grappling and real combat grappling. It's a place in which the martial artist can stop and control an aggressively intoxicated relative, friend, or coworker without causing injury or great pain."

—Loren W. Christensen, 8th dan black belt, author (www.lwcbooks.com)

"Responses to violence range from de-escalation and avoidance to less than lethal measures such as restraint and control techniques to inflicting serious bodily damage or even killing another human in self-defense. Physical techniques taught in martial art and self-defense programs also range from sport, to controlling an obnoxious relative or drunk (maybe an obnoxious drunk relative), to damaging and killing in all out combat. Kane and Wilder know these differences, and in *Dirty Ground*, they combine their years of traditional martial art training with their years of practical street experience to provide a guide to understanding and adapting your fighting techniques to the appropriate situation at hand. One technique does not fit all. Kane and Wilder show how you can adapt techniques to fit situations ranging from sport to drunk uncles to combat. Learn from this book and be better prepared for whatever response is required, whether that be sport, controlling people, or fighting for your life."

—Alain Burrese, J.D., former U.S. Army 2nd Infantry Division Scout Sniper School Instructor, author

"As you read the book remember this may be life altering. There is far too much in this volume to be able to do it justice in just a few words. Read it and take to heart what Lawrence and Kris are giving you from years of training and experience. There are a variety of levels of confrontation, some minor and easily avoided, others are real game changers. In more than 28 years of Law Enforcement and Corrections one thing is true, you can never be too prepared. On the job I cannot walk away from issues or confrontations. This book gives you options of what you can do from the lowest level (presence) to the highest level (deadly force) and all levels in between.

Along with the techniques is a very straight forward warning of what to expect after you have used force on someone. Depending on the level of force used and the situation there may be long lasting physical, mental, and emotional and possibly financial ramifications.

Work through the techniques given in the book and take a few that are appropriate for your level of skill and training and be prepared to use them if and when needed. As a private citizen it is best to avoid a confrontation if possible, but be prepared for those situations that are unavoidable. At the end of the day what matters to us all is the ability to go home safely to our family. The information and techniques in this book, if used with the intent and care intended, will us the greatest opportunity to meet that challenge."

—Mike McGinnis, Jail Administrative Officer

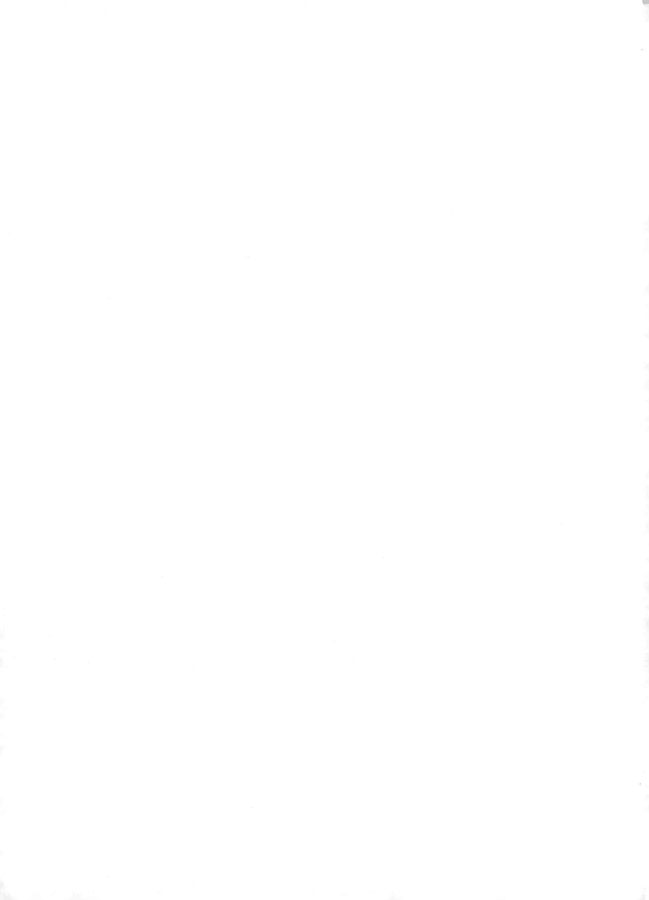

DIRTY GROUND

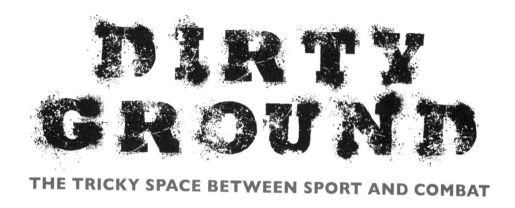

DIRTY GROUND

THE TRICKY SPACE BETWEEN SPORT AND COMBAT

KRIS WILDER AND LAWRENCE A. KANE

WITH ERIK McCRAY

YMAA Publication Center, Inc.
Wolfeboro NH USA

YMAA Publication Center, Inc.
PO Box 480
Wolfeboro, NH 03894
1-800-669-8892 • www.ymaa.com • info@ymaa.com

Print edition
ISBN-13: 978-1-59439-211-5   ISBN-10: 1-59439-211-0

Ebook edition
ISBN-13: 978-1-59439-261-0   ISBN-10: 1-59439-261-7

Cover design by Axie Breen
Editing by Susan Bullowa
Photos by Lawrence A. Kane
Illustrations by Kris Wilder

10   9   8   7   6   5   4   3   2   1

Publisher's Cataloging in Publication

Wilder, Kris.

Dirty ground : the tricky space between sport and
combat / Kris Wilder and Lawrence A. Kane ;
with Erik McCray. -- Wolfeboro, NH : YMAA Publication
Center, c2013.

p. ; cm.

ISBN: 978-1-59439-211-5 (print 13-digit);
1-59439-211-0 (print 10-digit); 978-1-59439-261-0
(ebk 13-digit); 1-59439-261-7 (ebk 10-digit)

Includes bibliographical references and index.

Summary: This book addresses the gap in martial arts training between sport and combat techniques:
that is when you need to control a person without severly injuring him (or her). Techniques in this space are
called 'drunkle'. The authors analyze 30 fundamental strikes, kicks and locks, and present 12 well-known sport
competition forms modified for each of the three vital environments: sport, drunkle, and combat.--Publisher.

1. Martial arts--Handbooks, manuals, etc.
2. Self-defense--Handbooks, manuals, etc.
3. Combat--Handbooks, manuals, etc. 4. Hand-to-hand fighting--Handbooks, manuals, etc. 5. Violence-
-Prevention--Handbooks, manuals, etc. 6. Assault and battery--Prevention--Handbooks, manuals, etc. I. Kane,
Lawrence A. (Lawrence Alan) II. McCray, Erik. III. Title.

GV1112 .W55 2013   2013932353

796.8/071--dc23   1305

Warning: While self-defense is legal, fighting is illegal. If you don't know the difference you'll go to jail because you aren't defending yourself. You are fighting—or worse. Readers are encouraged to be aware of all appropriate local and national laws relating to self-defense, reasonable force, and the use of weaponry, and act in accordance with all applicable laws at all times. Understand that while legal definitions and interpretations are generally uniform, there are small—but very important—differences from state to state and even city to city. To stay out of jail, you need to know these differences. Neither the authors nor the publisher assumes any responsibility for the use or misuse of information contained in this book.

Nothing in this document constitutes a legal opinion nor should any of its contents be treated as such. While the authors believe that everything herein is accurate, any questions regarding specific self-defense situations, legal liability, and/or interpretation of federal, state, or local laws should always be addressed by an attorney at law. This text relies on public news sources to gather information on various crimes and criminals described herein. While news reports of such incidences are generally accurate, they are on occasion incomplete or incorrect. Consequently, all suspects should be considered innocent until proven guilty in a court of law.

When it comes to martial arts, self-defense, and related topics, no text, no matter how well written, can substitute for professional, hands-on instruction. **These materials should be used for academic study only.**

Printed in Canada

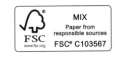

Table of Contents

Dedication

As you train in the martial arts—the hours, days, months, and years you log in pursuit of the craft—you come in contact with thousands of people: martial arts practitioners and instructors, some competent and some incompetent; it would be impossible for any martial artist who has trained any length of time to list all of those who have influenced them and shared their art.

One person who gets too little credit for the work he has done in the field of judo is Kenji Yamada. Born an American citizen, raised in Japan, and interned during World War II, his unassuming dogged determination and commitment to the art of judo brought him two United States grand championships in the 1950s and the admiration of countless students, the authors among them. A person whose teaching methods can only be described as "old school," his commitment to the art of judo bettered countless thousands of lives.

Acknowledgments

Thanking your parents and the role that they have played raising you to adulthood has become almost commonplace. Nonetheless, any work we produced that did not include an acknowledgment of the appreciation of our parents for their steadfast support and keen grasp on the challenges that face young men would be negligent. Without their guidance, we would certainly be lesser persons.

We have been fortunate to work with several publishers. Of them all, one stands above the rest: David Ripianzi from YMAA Publication Center. In a world that seems to consistently spin out of control, people of integrity and vision are rare. David not only has that combination, but he's also one heck of a good guy. We consider ourselves fortunate to be associated with YMAA and the direction that David brings to every project.

Foreword—by Rory Miller

If you fight, you fight for a goal and you fight in an environment. That is almost too obvious to write, but sometimes things need to be put into words or you lose track of obvious truths. When you lose track of obvious truths, you start to believe that a particular system, technique, or strategy is "right" when it is good only in a specific environment and aimed only at one of many possible goals.

I'll wager that any martial art you might study has a high degree of efficiency, that is, in the environment from which it evolved and when used to achieve the goal the system defined as the win.

Think about this: Modern *jujitsu*, think Brazilian *jiu-jitsu* (BJJ), is highly efficient, but doesn't look much like old, say pre-1650 Japanese *jujutsu* (JJJ). Old school JJJ doesn't have a lot of submissions and doesn't believe in spending much time working an opponent. Those strategies didn't make sense on a medieval battlefield where two guys grappling on the ground were easy kills for the spearmen on either side.

If the geniuses who founded BJJ (and I'm not talking about the people trying to retrofit it to fit the modern law enforcement or military "market") had lived in a time and place where the battlefield was the testing ground and a spear in the back was the penalty for "delay of game," the system would have looked much different. I bet it still would have been very efficient.

There are environmental factors in training as well. A system that takes a "lifetime to master" didn't have much utility to someone who was going into battle as soon as he reached puberty, and did "lifetime to master" mean the same thing, or even get said when the life expectancy was in the low 20s?

Modern systems designed for military recruits—young men full of testosterone and at peak fitness—don't require the same degree of efficiency as a system designed to protect the old and vulnerable from assault. Further, as battle changed over the centuries from a bloody hand-to-hand melee to a bloody technology-driven firefight, it made less and less sense to spend precious training time on unarmed fighting.

And one more point, from the environmental side: many of our martial arts systems predate the concept of self-defense law. In a world without effective police and courts, vengeance and the destruction of any serious threat made sense. The logical 1800 Okinawan solution to being attacked may risk prison time today. The world has changed.

In this book, Wilder and Kane talk about the other dimension: how goals, what you are fighting for, change every element of how you fight.

In a sport environment you want to win, quickly and decisively, but with solid assurance that your opponent will be able to get back up and play again tomorrow. In a combat situation you want to win quickly and decisively, but with solid assurance that your foe cannot get up and re-engage until you are long gone, if ever.

If you are trying to get the car keys from your drunken uncle or breaking up a family fight, not only do you want zero injury, but you are not dealing with trained competitors and the person you are throwing, locking, or striking may not be capable of protecting him or herself. That puts the responsibility for both the throw AND the fall entirely on you.

Self-defense is the biggest change and the hardest of all—you must make your technique work whatever your goal sometimes to incapacitate the threat, sometimes simply to escape—when you have already taken damage, your structure is compromised and applied against a threat who is bigger, stronger, and has complete tactical advantage. That's the baseline for surviving assault and it is a world beyond the difference between sport and war.

Simple changes in goals profoundly change how you prioritize your choices (weapons are unacceptable when drunk-wrangling but the first choice in combat) and how you execute your technique (at least one *koryu* version of *osoto gari* collapses the trachea, blows out the knees, and dumps the threat on his back).

What the authors have done in this book is simply to give you a taste. Don't try to memorize the differences in application between a technique used on an enemy and a drunk. Try to understand the differences and then take a hard look at your own training. Knowing that there is a difference between submitting an opponent and disabling an enemy is not the same as practicing the difference, nor is it a guarantee that you can switch to the appropriate mindset at the right time.

If you are preserving a quick-killing soldier's art from the old days, what must be modified to handle someone you don't wish to hurt? What must you learn to bring it in line with a legal environment the founders never imagined?

Studying one thing is not, and never can be, studying everything.

Train hard. Pay attention. Ask questions. Do your best to always be clear about what you are really doing and why.

Rory Miller is the author of *Meditations on Violence, Violence: A Writer's Guide, Facing Violence*, and *Force Decisions*, among others, and co-author (with Lawrence Kane) of *Scaling Force*. His writings have also been featured in Loren Christensen's *Fighter's Fact Book 2*, Kane/Wilder's *The Little Black Book of Violence*, and *The Way to Black Belt*. He has been studying martial arts since 1981. Though he started in competitive martial sports, earning college varsities in judo and fencing, he found his martial "home" in the early Tokugawa-era battlefield system of *Sosuishi-ryu kumi uchi* (*jujutsu*).

A veteran corrections officer and Corrections Emergency Response Team (CERT) leader, Rory has hands-on experience in hundreds of violent altercations. He has designed and taught courses for law enforcement agencies including confrontational simulations, uncontrolled environments, crisis communications with the mentally ill, CERT operations and planning, defensive tactics, and use of force policy. His training also includes witness protection, close-quarters handgun, Americans for Effective Law Enforcement (AELE) discipline and internal investigations, hostage negotiations, and survival and integrated use of force.

He recently spent a year in Iraq helping the government there develop its prison management system. Rory currently teaches seminars on violence internationally, and in partnership with Marc MacYoung has developed Conflict Communications, a definitive resource for understanding and controlling conflict. Rory's website is www.chirontraining.com. He lives near Portland, Oregon.

Foreword—by Marc MacYoung

The last time I found myself looking down the barrel of a cop's gun, I was kneeling on some guy's head.

In the officer's defense, it was the middle night in a bad part of town, we were out on the sidewalk and there were two of us on top of this guy. So his pointing a pistol at us was an understandable reaction.

The nice policemen suggested that I and my partner might want to stop what we were doing and allow the other gentleman to get up. I held up my hands and said, "I will comply! But this guy is on the fight and, if we let him go, there's a good chance he'll attack us again."

Still, the officer was adamant about us letting the li'l feller go. While we were discussing his release, two more police cars arrived. We stepped back and the guy popped up like a jack-in-the-box from hell. We were quickly separated into two groups by the officers and questioned. As should be the case, we were facing the officer interviewing us with our backs to the other individual involved.

We told our story: who we were, where we worked, that this intoxicated individual had attacked two customers attempting to enter the business. We'd come to their assistance. He had a death grip on one of the customer's shirt and I'd used a knife to cut it, so they could jump in their car and leave the scrap of cloth that was still lying on the sidewalk). We'd waited until they had left, then we let him up. When we did so, he'd attacked us. Once again we'd put him down in a controlled manner and were trying to talk him down when the officer had arrived.

The officer looked at me and asked, "Did you hit him?"

"No sir. I did a prescribed takedown to control him without injury. We never struck him, just controlled him so he couldn't hurt us or the others."

About then the other party decided to offer a suggestion to a female police officer. Not only was the suggestion not polite, but it was loud too. As a final point, he called her a name. Women generally do not like being referred to as that particular part of their anatomy.

The officer in front of us blinked when he heard this. He quietly said, "You two can go." We politely thanked the officer and returned to the business. We looked over to see our old friend now had new friends—who were also kneeling on his head.

This story exemplifies many different and important points about a violent encounter. First of all, odds are good you will be dealing with the police.

Second, there was a potentially deadly weapon present. It wasn't used on anyone. It was used to cut cloth to let someone escape and then it was put away. Could I have slashed his arm? Yes. And I would have gone to prison for assault with a deadly weapon because it wasn't necessary.

Third, this situation wasn't self-defense. Nor was it a "fight" to win, dominate, or prove whose pee-pee was bigger, teach someone a lesson, or punish him. None of the normal definitions people commonly banter around in the martial arts applied to this situation.

Fourth, it was a use-of-force situation with a clearly defined goal, tactics, and integrated with verbal communication. "We don't want to hurt you. If you calm down, we'll let you up."

Fifth, not only would punching the guy have been inappropriate, but it would have gotten us arrested. That question about whether or not we had hit him was a trap to get us to admit excessive force. But that's not as important as knowing that use of force is a "Goldilocks and the Three Bears" issue. This one is too little. This one is too much. This one is just right.

Sixth, our calm, professional, and cooperative demeanor—as we articulated the facts of the situation—is what kept us from getting arrested. This, even though the situation had started with us looking down the barrel of a pistol. Had we jumped up and down, howled, screamed, made accusations, and insulted the other guy, we would have ended up, like him, down on the ground with someone kneeling on our heads.

Dirty Ground won't teach you how to deal with the police. What it will do is help you understand use of force choices and pick a response that is both better for the task at hand and more defensible. That's a pretty important thing to know. It's also a gaping hole in most martial arts AND so-called "self-defense" training.

Simply stated, despite fantasies about muggers and drugged up bikers jumping you, most violence happens between people who know each other. Yes, it could be a fight or it could just as likely be something else. What? Having to drag a drunken friend who's out of line from a party, or your mother comes to you at a family reunion and says, "Your uncle Albert is drunk again; you're a martial artist; go deal with him." These are the everyday realities of how violence actually happens. Realities ignored by most training.

You can't punch Drunken Uncle Albert without getting Aunt Betty mad at you. If you do, odds are good he'll punch you back and you'll be in a fight. This doesn't look good either with your family members or the police when you try to convince them you weren't fighting. Punching him also doesn't win you points with your drunken friend when he sobers up.

Controlling someone without hurting him is exactly what grappling is best for. It is, by definition, a dominance and submission game without injury. You can defend your actions to the police a lot better by grappling with someone who is acting up a lot better than you can by punching him out.

This is why *Dirty Ground* is such an important book. It looks at the actual application of grappling in that context instead of the fantasy of "self-defense" or the restrictions of the ring.

Growing up on gang-infested streets not only gave Marc MacYoung his street name "Animal," but also extensive firsthand experience about what does and does not work for self-defense. Over the years, he has held a number of dangerous occupations including director of a correctional institute, bodyguard, and bouncer. He was first shot at when he was 15 years old and has since survived multiple attempts on his life, including professional contracts. He has studied a variety of martial arts since childhood, teaching experience-based self-defense to police, military, civilians, and martial artists around the world. He has written dozens of books and produced numerous DVDs covering all aspects of this field. Oh yeah, he's also been seen hanging out with Rory Miller recently.

Why This Book?

This book was written to address an important gap that exists in martial arts. The tricky issue is the space in between sport and combat, as well as the chasm that separates these two extremes. In order of severity, we call these three environments, sport, drunkle, and combat. Drunkle is a combination of the words "drunk" and "uncle," referring to situations in which you need to control a person without severely injuring him (or her). Understanding these environments is vital because what is considered appropriate use of force is codified in law, yet interpreted in the public arena. Actions that do not accommodate these rules can have severe repercussions. Techniques must be adapted to best fit the situation you find yourself in.

While the differences between sport and combat are somewhat intuitive, it is important to clarify exactly what we mean by these terms. The *Merriam-Webster Dictionary* defines sport as: "Physical activity engaged in for pleasure," whereas combat is described as coming from Anglo-French roots, *combate*, to attack, or fight, and from Latin, *battuere*, "to beat." Okay, so we can regurgitate definitions out of a dictionary, big fat freaking deal. Let's cut to the chase—sports are competitions, stuff you want to win that are specifically designed so that competitors don't get seriously hurt. Combat, on the other hand, is designed to kill people, break things, and blow stuff up. They're worlds apart.

Martial sports, judo, boxing, wrestling, *jujitsu*, *sumo*, mixed martial arts (MMA), and the like are a fantastic means of training one's body and mind, even of forging one's spirit. And as a sport, each one of these has rules, built-in faults that allow for intense physical contact while minimizing the threat of life and limb. An example of this is "the rabbit punch." The rabbit punch, usually a swinging hook punch to the back of an opponent's head while in a clinch, is illegal in boxing, MMA, and many other sports. An important reason for banning this technique is that it attacks the connection between the base of the skull and the spinal column. In acupuncture, this location is called Gall Bladder 20, and in Western medicine it is C1 (Cervical 1). To the medieval executioner, it was the general area where the ax would fall to sever a condemned person's head from his body. A severe blow to this area from a practitioner's fist can have the same consequence as that headsman's ax, minus the messy decapitation—it can kill.

Another example is that in tournament judo, MMA, and the like, you pin your opponent face up so that he can have a fighting chance to continue the match. Law enforcement officers oftentimes use the same techniques, yet they pin the suspect face down so that he cannot put up much of a fight while being handcuffed. In this example, the same application is applied in a different environment. Safety rules can change the technique, the application, or the context.

Without these rules, a sport becomes combat; with these rules combat becomes sport.

If you are a citizen, your role in society (legally, if not morally and ethically as well) is to get away from violence, to escape. Law enforcement officers have a duty to act, they must become involved, but unless you've got a badge, you don't have to. Unless the violence is directed at you and you cannot avoid it. Depending on the circumstances, you might then have to cripple or kill another person in order to escape from harm. Nevertheless, your purpose is not to arrest the other guy, beat him down, teach him a lesson, or otherwise "win" the encounter.

As a competitor in sports, on the other hand, your role *is* to win. The rules are designed to allow you to intensify your actions with minimal risk of injury. You are able to use one hundred percent of your physical ability because you are assured, due to safety gear, rules, referees, and whatnot, that there is only a very slight opportunity for you or your opponent to experience life-altering events because of your actions. This intensification of action, with safety precautions, gives you a powerful and competitive experience.

If you are a soldier, your job is to convert people from living to dead. Sure, you do other things as well, but that's the bottom line. Nevertheless, you need to practice killing people without actually doing it. Consequently rules and specially designed safety equipment are used to reduce the intensity of your actions so that you may train for war with some level of safety. Like referees, drill instructors oversee the action and enforce the rules... until you hit the battlefield and use what you have learned to defeat the enemy.

Commonly four areas are addressed to limit damage: reduction of angle, intensity, weapon, or striking area. These are the keys to creating safe training/competition.

That all takes place in a practice hall, training course, or tournament ring, yet from a certain perspective, the same thing happens on the street. How you choose the angle, intensity, weapon, and striking areas will, in large part, affect the outcome. This is how sport and combat can overlap and is called the "critical point." This is the place where sport can become combat and where combat can become sport. The decisions you make determine which direction your engagement will take.

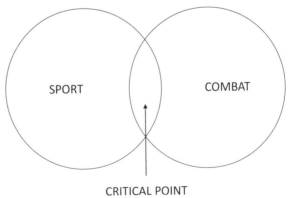

What You Will Find in This Book

How to end a fight at grappling distance, using the ancient tried-and-true three-point military concept of ground, clear, and insert.

Ground: Drive the opponent to the ground via any means necessary.

Clear: Open a space, clear their weapon, or take advantage of a space.

Insert: Insert your weapon into the cleared space.

You probably know that we're traditionalists, guys who study and teach martial arts that were historically designed to create cripples and corpses, so perhaps you also expect us to bag on "combative sports." Not gonna happen. These things have their place. The athletes who participate in them are tough, skilled, and in great shape. They just do something that's a little different than we do, or perhaps more accurately, have a different focus. Similarly, we're not going to get into which system is better, UFC, K1, Pride, or whatever… Who cares; it's pointless. Each form of sport has its rules and those rules are used for protection, securing victory, and ensuring continued participation and enjoyment by the participants and spectators alike. That's what matters.

The Origins of This Book

Look at it this way. If you were a *kobudoka* in ancient Okinawa with a *bo* staff, your intent clearly would not have been to spend fifteen minutes engaged with an armed adversary. Chances are good that you wouldn't be able to walk away from something like that, and even if you did you probably would have been busted up so badly that without modern medicine you'd have died within a week or two anyway. In combat, you don't want to engage your adversary for any significant length of time, it's too dangerous. You want to kill or disable him swiftly.

The same concept applies to modern times. With rifles, artillery, aircraft, and other weapons, you end the conflict by killing at a distance. In fact, the last major time the United States Army fixed bayonets to their rifles, effectively turning a long range weapon into a close-range weapon, and charged the enemy was during the Korean War on February 7, 1951. This assault was led by Lewis Lee Millett, Sr., who received a Medal of Honor for his heroism during the engagement. In war, more distance is much better. The key to successfully shooting down an enemy aircraft, for example, is to see the other guy before he sees you and put a missile up his tailpipe before he even knows you're there. Obviously, most of us aren't flying around in fighter jets, but hopefully you get the point.…

When you step onto the mat to engage an opponent in a grappling competition, the action is up close and personal. Matches take a really long time, the exact opposite strategy of what you would want in warfare. Heck, you can spend a full round in the guard or take two or three minutes trying to get an armbar, in part because the other guy's friends aren't circling around trying to kick your head in while you're doing it. While all these things take a great amount of skill and are important in their own right, their value diminishes in a combative situation. In the ring, you are not engaging an enemy at your preferred distance, on your terms, and ending the fight as expeditiously as possible.

You already know we're not going to get into the "this art form is better than that art form" argument. However, there are differences that matter. Those differences are determined by several factors, some of which include the health of the person, their body type, their mental state, and their level of training.

What Will Be Covered Here

The ancient concepts of battle will be revisited and renewed. Not ancient techniques but tried-and-true, battle-tested strategies that have been proven successful. Modern interpretations of these ancient concepts and strategies will be demonstrated and explored as form follows function—environments change, and so should martial arts. The moral implications of such combative actions will also be addressed briefly. Our goal is to make these concepts usable, not to pontificate.

The Challenges of This Book

Thankfully more people are involved in sports than in combat. There are more citizens than soldiers. So in the interest of accessibility, the sport aspect of grappling is used as an entry point as it is the most common experience. We have tried to put some context around the applications and even give y'all a little history lesson to prove our points. But, without exception, historical and contemporary greats have been left out of the discussion. These omissions are not an affront; they keep this book reasonable in size and focus.

We're style agnostic here, and we use techniques you've probably seen before, but what's shown are merely examples. There is no way we can be comprehensive in a single tome. By the time you finish, you will understand how common applications can be modified for sport, drunkle, and combat environments. Take the principles you learn and apply them to whatever style you study.

Who is This Book for?

While not everyone competes in tournaments, virtually anyone could find themselves in a situation where they face a combat or drunkle encounter. If you have studied a martial sport or practice a martial art to help keep yourself safe from violence, odds are good you've discovered a proclivity for either stand-up fighting or grappling. Given these predilections, here's how the materials apply.

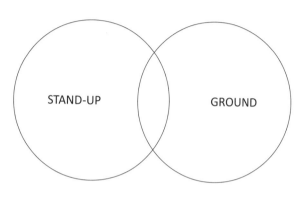

Stand-up Fighters

If you are a boxer, *karateka*, *taekwondo* practitioner, or some other type of stand-up fighter, this book is designed for you. The Ultimate Fighting Championship (UFC) is an excellent example of the cross-breeding of stand-up and ground techniques. Mixed martial arts demonstrate that skilled grapplers can use their expertise to overcome a stand-up fighter/striker who has limited ground experience. This is not a disparaging remark toward the stand-up fighter, nor an assertion of technical superiority for the ground fighter, merely a reflection of a moment in time, a fact.

MMA rules tend to give grapplers the upper hand in the ring in some ways, but let's face it, you need a broad skill set to survive on the street too. How many fights wind up on the ground? It's not the ninety percent that some people think, but it's certainly a lot of them. Could be the one you find yourself in… Think about how badly you will get hurt if you wind up in a situation for which you have no response. Stand-up fighters need a ground game too.

Grapplers

If you are a grappler, a person that spends a lot of time on his hands, knees, and back, then this book is also for you. *Ne-waza,* or groundwork, is a great form of training. It can produce a high level of grappling acuity that can be used in a stress situation. It's something you need to experience to become good at. But, if you use sporting applications in a life-or-death struggle then, well, let's just say it won't end well… On the street, you need to *think* like a striker even when you're applying grappling techniques.

Whether you use groundwork or stand-up, in a real fight you need to have an "end it now" attitude. For grapplers, this book will help you isolate your skills so as to take advantage of a situation and finish a conflict quickly. For stand-up fighters, you will discover that the ground oftentimes hits harder than you can. You will learn ways to take advantage of that too.

Let's face it; you cannot learn the applications shown here without spending significant time on the mat. Find a good instructor and practice. Learning how to differentiate tactics and techniques you already know for sport, drunkle, or all-out combat will take that practice to a whole new level.

Sport versus Combat

It was the first time I'd ever made it to the finals. Win and I'd take home the first place trophy; lose and it'd still be a pretty cool piece of hardware. I'd come in third a couple of times, but the little statues weren't nearly as prestigious as the big ones. And I really, really wanted to earn one of the big ones.

Jumping up and down a couple times I loosened my shoulders and then twisted my head to each side to pop my neck. I stepped up to the line thinking, "Okay, I am so ready for this."

"Hajime!"

The referee dropped his hand and we surged forward, working our grips and jockeying for position. I got a hold of him, crashed forward, and attempted an osoto gari foot sweep. I had pretty good timing, but didn't get enough hip rotation so it failed. Before I could move to something else, he countered with the same technique.

I landed awkwardly, but on my side, taking him down with me so he didn't score a point. But he did get a hold of my lapel, simultaneously wrapping his legs around my waist. I drove an elbow down, made a wedge, and tried to twist away. I was vaguely aware of pressure on my neck, but didn't really think anything about it… until I woke up.

Damn, he'd choked me out. How the hell did that happen so fast?

At least I'd get a shot at a rematch next month…

The attributes of sports are:

- Pageantry
- Timelines
- Scoring
- Competitors able to compete again after the match

Combat differs in that it is an open and armed conflict with intent to kill the enemy and/or destroy their infrastructure. There may be some level of pageantry, but rarely a timeline, and "scoring" is based on killing the opponent and/or breaking his will to continue to fight. Many participants do not survive. Those who do are often never the same again, requiring lengthy rehabilitation for serious physical or, in some cases, mental injuries.

Think of it this way. If a 250-pound tattooed steroid freak tells you to show up at a certain place and time where he's going to beat the crap out of you, you could react in couple different ways. If you're thinking sport, you show up at the venue, strap on the gloves, and have a go at it. If you're thinking combat, you wait in ambush and blow his head off when he arrives. Or bomb the building once he goes inside.

Sport rules can be anything from how you can use your hands to what kind of equipment is required. There is a beginning, middle, and an end to the sporting event, with timelines known to all participants ahead of time. The rules are designed to ensure that the participants have a level of safety that brings an ability to participate again at a later date, sometimes again that same day.

Another aspect of sport is the pageantry that is associated with the event. There can be all sorts of formal pageantry, everything from uniforms and titles to ceremonies prior to the sporting event, observances after the sporting event, or even rites performed in the middle. You can think of it in terms of a football game in the United States with the singing of the national anthem, the halftime entertainment, and then the awarding of a trophy at the end of a particularly significant game.

Sport rules also support a form of competition that keeps the spectator engaged, so they may enjoy the competition as much as the participants. Typically, these rules include leveling the playing field to increase the chances of an exciting event. A spectator isn't going enjoy watching a 250-pound *judoka* take on a 115-pound opponent any more than he will like watching a professional football team play against a bunch of high school athletes. We all know that the smaller person has little chance under sports rules that take truly dangerous techniques out of play. It is just a matter of time before the bigger competitor falls on the smaller competitor and the match is over.

Specialization exists in every sport. An example of specialization is the designated hitter in the American League of Major League Baseball. This player does nothing but bat the ball. Unlike everyone else on the team, he does not play a position on the field. In American football, an offensive tackle may weigh upward of 300 pounds. His job is to stop people from getting past him, people who tend to match up favorably in size and speed. Compare this to the average wide receiver who weighs in at 200 pounds or less. The smaller, faster receiver's job is to get away from other players, catch the ball, and travel as far down the field as he can before being tackled. Sporting rules allow for specialization, and in that specialization, comes the context in which to enjoy the event.

It's not that warriors don't specialize, they often do, but that both teams have the same mix of specializations (e.g., quarterbacks, receivers, kickers, punters, linebackers, safeties, and the like).

The time line is one of the biggest separators between sport and combat. Although not all sports use a clock (like baseball), the majority of sports use some kind of a timer. Those that don't count periods such as rounds or innings instead. The reason for this is that a clock provides an external pressure determining the intensity of play. Players and coaches have little control over the clock other than a few timeouts. In combat, the battle rages until one side or the other gives up or moves for a political solution (we're not aware of any wars in the last few centuries where one side completely wiped out the other).

The assumption is that in combat and war there are no rules of engagement but in reality there are. A good example would be the Geneva Protocol to the Hague Convention. Signed in 1925, it involved, among other things, permanently banning all forms of chemical and biological warfare. This protocol came about after World War I where the use of mustard gas and other similar chemicals not only killed thousands upon thousands of soldiers but also left many of them blinded and maimed.

Approximately seven years after World War I, more rules of warfare were put in place, including the illegality of the triangle-shaped blade on a bayonet. This prohibition was adopted because the resulting triangular wound was very difficult for a surgeon or field doctor to suture. The intent of the triangle-shaped blade was to create a wound that remained open as long as possible. If the wound site became infected, the injured soldier would not only be incapacitated but would eventually die from that contagion.

These are two examples of rules of combat. Unlike sport, there is no clock in war and combat is about battles of dominance, submission, and attrition. In the simplest terms, victory is ensured by breaking more of the other combatant's things (e.g., buildings, roads, infrastructure, and equipment) and killing more of their people than they kill of yours so that they will eventually give up. Media and political pressure play an important role.

Drunkles, Druggles, Dysfunctional Relatives, and Whacked-Out Friends

It was my turn to watch the door. Everyone at the party had left their keys on a pegboard and I wasn't supposed to give them back unless the person was sober enough to drive. About midnight Ron staggered up to me and demanded his keys. He was hammered, so I told him no, something along the lines of, "You've got to sober up first, man."

Well, he wasn't having any of that. He lunged for the keys. I got there first, grabbed them off the board, and twisted away from him. I told him no again, but he kept coming. He was bigger than me, and a serious asshole when drunk, but he was my fraternity brother and I wasn't about to let him kill himself or someone else driving home. Unfortunately, the other guys just thought it was funny. They were no help. Until he grabbed me by the throat and tried choking me.

I drove my knee into his stomach. It wasn't much of a blow but it did force him back. As he lunged again I pivoted and hit him in the base of the jaw as hard as I could. Much to my surprise he crumbled to the ground. It was the first time I'd ever knocked anyone out. Thankfully, the next morning he didn't remember who'd hit him…

A couple months later it got worse. Our frat was one of the only ones in the U-District with a parking lot. Space being at a premium, that land was worth more than our house and everything in it combined. There was enough room on the street to accommodate most who lived in the area—but not nearly enough for townies, party guests, and the like so guys from nearby houses kept parking on our property. Despite the warnings, tow trucks, and even a few fistfights, they'd been doing it all semester. Then a couple guys from the fraternity across the street keyed a few of our vehicles in retaliation.

That didn't go over very well. Within minutes, some seventy of us were brawling in the street, Ron leading the charge.

Being somewhat smarter, or at least more sober than most, I chose not to participate. I was watching the ruckus from the front yard when Ron stumbled past, nose gushing blood, and disappeared into the house. Thinking he was hurt more seriously than a busted nose to have left the fight like that, I turned and followed him in, but I couldn't find him on the main floor. As I passed the stairs leading to our rooms above, I spotted him heading back down, murder in his eyes and a rifle in his hands. Holy shit! I didn't even know he had a gun, let alone would be stupid enough to bring one to a fistfight!

I bolted to the front, grabbed three other guys who had also been watching the scrap in the street, and blocked the door. We tried to talk some sense into him but Ron was too enraged to listen. He kept right on moving, shoving his way past us. We undoubtedly underestimated the true danger we faced. I know that I certainly did, but there was no way in hell I was about to let him out that door. I dove for his knees, striking with my shoulder and wrapping him up like I'd learned to tackle playing football. It didn't work (did I mention that Ron was a hell of a lot bigger and stronger than me?). After a slight hesitation, probably all of a half second but it seemed a couple decades longer at the time, the other guys jumped in as well.

The four of us managed to wrestle him to the ground, wrench the rifle out of his hands, and sit on him until he calmed down. And, thankfully, the gun didn't discharge during the altercation. If we had not intervened, I'm certain that Ron would have killed someone over scratched paint.

Drunkle is an important concept when choosing the right way to respond to any given situation, so it merits a bit more detail. Drunkles do not necessarily have to be your intoxicated, socially awkward uncle, or even your relative. They can be your loud-mouthed buddy trying to pick a fight he's about to lose or drag you unwillingly into, your best friend coming off a bad drug trip (which would make him a druggle technically), your teenage son throwing things and breaking furniture in a hormonal rage, your suicidal sister with a bottle of champagne and a handful of sleeping pills, or even your idiot fraternity brother with a gun.

These are all situations where you know the other guy (or gal) needs some type of adult "spanking," which is both warranted and necessary, and you're the one who has to mete out that punishment, or "time out" or whatever you want to call it. The key is that you are neither participating in a sports competition nor engaging in combat to defend your life or that of a loved one, but rather you are squarely in that shadow region that lies in the middle of those two extremes. Characteristics of a drunkle situation include:

- You are related to, or friends with, the drunkle.
- You feel it is appropriate to intervene in order to stop the drunkle from doing something stupid, harmful, or violent.

- You would prefer that the drunkle not to be arrested for his actions, hence unwilling to simply stand by and let someone with authority intervene (or there's no time for that).

- Because of your relationship with the drunkle, you believe that it is unlikely that he would press charges against you once sobered up (assuming you are able to control him without breaking him).

- You don't mind so much if the drunkle is hurt (pain) by what you must do, but you strive to avoid causing any serious or lasting injury (damage).

Sometimes resolution is as simple as a light touch on the drunkle's shoulder (or a swift kick to his shin) to warn him against whatever he is about to do. Other times dragging him away from the problem and giving a stern lecture can be effective. Oftentimes, however, these situations require forcefully putting the drunkle on the ground and holding him there for a while. That's one of the best ways to contain a bad situation without injuring anyone. When it works.

You do need a certain level of skill and sobriety to pull it off. The bad news is that such actions can be physically dangerous for both of you (not to mention your relationship). Your edge in skill and sobriety makes you responsible (ethically at least) both for the technique you choose to put him on the ground as well for the results of his landing there. If you do it right, you can usually get away with it. Physically. If you're lucky he may even thank you for what you did the next day too (but don't count on that).

There is one other potential piece of good news as well. There's no guarantee, of course, but law enforcement officers tend to be pretty understanding of these situations too. It won't look good when they first see you sitting on the drunkle, but oftentimes they will cut you some slack once they learn what took place. If you are sober, didn't actually hit the drunkle (or at least did not draw blood), and are able to explain the situation articulately, you are likely to avoid being arrested (or at least being prosecuted).

As mentioned previously, this isn't sport, but it isn't combat either. It's that wide gap in between where much social violence occurs. You don't want or need to kill the other guy or put him in the hospital. In fact, you probably don't even want to bust him up (well maybe you *want* to, but prudence dictates that you shouldn't). Most times you're hoping to maintain an ongoing relationship with him. Consequently, successful resolution means that everyone goes home safely afterward with nothing worse than hurt feelings and a few bruises.

The Morality of Fighting

I was sitting in my living room watching television when I heard a loud crash followed by the sound of breaking glass outside. Looking out a window I saw a teenage saggy pants, 'banger wannabe walking up the street with an aluminum baseball bat in his hands. Every time he passed a car he'd take out a side-view mirror, headlight, or window with a swing. Realizing there was only a dozen feet between this hooligan and my car I dashed out the door to confront him.

"What the hell are you doing?" Not the best way to deescalate a bad situation, but in the spur of the moment I couldn't think of anything else to say.

"Fuck you!"

"Stay away from my car."

"What part of 'fuck you,' don't you understand asshole!"

"Put down the bat."

"Like hell. I'm gonna shove it up your ass until you choke!"

Well, that wasn't going very well. I considered drawing my gun when he swung at me a few heartbeats later, but punk was much younger than I was and I didn't think that blowing his head off would play well in the press despite the fact that he was armed with a bat. Besides, for a martial arts instructor and firearms expert, I really am a pretty non-violent guy. I had enough experience with weapons that I thought I had a pretty good idea of what to do.

In my sword training, there was a tandem drill that taught us how to use range and angle to avoid a strike. As the blow comes toward us, we shift slightly out of range to keep from being hit, then follow the weapon back in to counterattack before it can be redirected. Although it is a sword-to-sword drill, I figured that the same principles would apply to an unarmed confrontation against a bat as well.

Assuming I could use the same technique to disarm this kid without either of us getting hurt, I prepared to do so. Unfortunately, he wasn't on the same lesson plan. As I shifted out of range, he let go of the bat, something I'd never seen done with a sword. People only throw their weapons in the movies. Or so I'd thought. Unfortunately the bat flew a short distance through the air and rapped me across the head and shoulder with stunning force.

Before I realized what had happened I was on the ground. I don't remember falling, yet once I hit the ground I still had the presence of mind to scissor his legs, knocking him down before he could do anything worse. I followed up by grabbing a hold of one of his feet, pulling him in, and simultaneously kicking him in the 'nads to end the fight. I was still seeing stars when he staggered to his feet and lurched away.

Pretty cool, huh? Heroic even. The badass black belt gets whomped upside the head with an aluminum baseball bat yet perseveres and manages to take out the bad guy. Yeah, right. It was one of the most dumbass things I've ever done. Seriously.

Here's the deal: whenever you go hands-on there are consequences. In this case it was mild concussion and a bunch of scrapes and bruises. Not too bad. I've had worse in training, but it could very easily have been catastrophic. What if he'd staved in my skull with the bat? What if the he'd hit his head on the curb when I knocked him down? Or broke his neck during the fall? Or, what if the cops had decided to push the issue when they showed up half an hour later and referred me for prosecution…

"What?" you ask. "Why would they prosecute me? I was the good guy!" Well, not really. The kid with the bat wasn't the only one who had broken the law… (And I can say that now since the Statute of Limitations has run its course.)

Okay, we've covered the drunkle, so now let's take a hard look at fighting and self-defense. While this brief overview is no substitute for a holistic understanding of the law and a competent attorney to represent you in court, the following information may keep you from needing to hire one. Maybe. Consider it a place to start.

Self-defense is an affirmative plea. That's a huge freaking deal. It means that instead of the burden of proof resting with the prosecutor, you being innocent until proven guilty and all that, it shifts that burden to you. In other words, you tell the judge and jury that you did it ("it" being killing, maiming, assaulting, or whatever the other guy), but that you had a really damn good excuse.

"Yup, I killed him your honor. But he tried to kill me first…" It's actually a hell of a lot more complicated than that, but you get the idea.

Under the right circumstances, you have a legitimate excuse for breaking the law and will not be held criminally liable for your actions, which doesn't mean you won't subsequently be sued in civil court. While taking a life is obviously illegal, the competing harm (or urgent necessity as they call it in some jurisdictions) of saving your own life outweighs the harm you did to your attacker. If he initiated the confrontation and if you did nothing to escalate it. You have to be completely innocent. And you have to be able to prove it in court.

Generally, to successfully prove your case you must show evidence that:

1. The harm you sought to avoid outweighed the danger of the prohibited conduct you were charged with. *In the example above, kicking a guy in the balls is less dangerous than being whacked with a bat, but proved effective anyway. Technically, the bat is just as deadly as a gun in close quarters, so I would probably have been justified in shooting him to stave off a deadly threat. Protecting my life without taking his; it's all good baby.*

2. You had no reasonable alternative but to engage in the prohibited conduct in order to avoid that harm. *At the moment of the fight, this criterion was true, but in the aforementioned example staying in the living room, picking up the phone, and calling the police to deal with the punk would have precluded the necessity for fighting. And, if you've got time to think about the legal and public relations ramifications of what you're about to do, odds are you aren't in immediate danger. Flunked this one big time!*

3. You stopped doing the prohibited conduct as soon as the danger passed. *Once the teenager was no longer a threat, the countervailing force ceased. I stopped hitting him and even let him walk away when he chose to disengage. We're good here.*

4. You did not create the danger you sought to avoid. *Another failure; the confrontation was easily avoidable. If I'd shot him, I'd probably still be in jail. Thankfully it all turned out all right, but so far as decision-making goes this one sucks blocky nuts for me...*

So, how do you know you're doing the right thing? At the simplest level, if the following four criteria are all met you have a pretty good legal case for taking physical action to defend yourself: (1) ability, (2) opportunity, (3) jeopardy, and (4) preclusion. This is commonly known as AOJP. If any one (or more) of these conditions are absent, you are on shaky legal ground. That will virtually always cost you.

Ability

Ability means that an attacker has both the physical as well as practical ability to seriously injure, maim, or kill you. This may include the use of fists and feet as well as the application of conventional or improvised weapons such as knives, guns, bottles, baseball bats, or similar instruments. It also includes the physical ability to wield said weapon (or fists or feet for that matter) in a manner that can actually injure you. A small child with a baseball bat does not have the same ability to cause harm as the street punk swinging the same weapon.

Opportunity

While your attacker may have the ability to harm you, his ability does not necessarily mean that he also has the immediate opportunity to do so. Your life and well-being (or that of someone you need to protect) must be in clear and present danger before you can legally respond with a significant level of physical force. For example, a bad guy with a knife has the ability to kill you only so long as he is also within striking range of the weapon or can quickly move into the appropriate distance from which to initiate his attack. A physical barrier such as a chain link fence may protect you from a knife-wielder but not an assailant armed with a gun, so opportunity relates not only to the attacker and the weapon, but also to the environment within which they are deployed as well.

Jeopardy

Jeopardy or "imminent jeopardy," as the law sometimes requires, relates to the specifics of the situation. Any reasonable person in a similar situation should feel in fear for his life. This is a legal attempt to distinguish between a truly hazardous situation and one that is only potentially dangerous. While you are not expected to be able to read a threat's mind, you certainly should be able to ascertain his intent from his outward appearance, demeanor, and actions. Someone shouting, "I'm going to kill you" while walking away is probably not an immediate threat even though he may very well come back with a weapon or a group of friends later and become one should you stick around long enough. Someone shouting, "I love you" while lunging toward you with a knife, on the other hand, most likely is an imminent threat.

Preclusion

Even when the ability, opportunity, and jeopardy criteria are satisfied, you must still have no other safe alternatives other than physical force before engaging an opponent in combat. If you could have stayed safely behind a locked door and dialed 9-1-1 yet chose to step outside and challenge the bad guy, you have blown this rule. Similarly, if you can run or retreat from harm's way without further endangering yourself, these criteria have not been met. In some jurisdictions, there is no requirement to retreat when attacked in your home or, in some cases, your place of business. This is frequently referred to as "castle" laws. Regardless, it is prudent to retreat whenever you have the ability to do so safely. After all, it is impossible for the other guy to hurt you if you're not there.

Okay, so AOJP can help you know when it's prudent to go hands-on, but the next million dollar question is how much force to use. Use too little and you might not survive, too much and you'll likely wind up in jail.

Levels of Force

During the escalation process there are several force options that can help stave off violence: presence, voice, touch, empty-hand restraint, less-lethal force, and lethal force. This continuum is similar to the approach codified by many police departments. The first three levels can potentially prevent violence before it begins, the fourth may be used proactively as an opponent prepares to strike, and the last two generally take place after you have already been attacked (usually when you're losing). You do not have to move from one level to another, but rather need to enter at the appropriate level for the threat you face, and adjust appropriately as the tactical situation warrants.

1. Presence—Use of techniques designed to stave off violence via posture or body language that warns adversaries of your readiness and ability to act, or body language that poses no threat to another's ego.

2. Voice—Use of techniques designed to verbally de-escalate conflict before physical methods become necessary.

3. Touch—Use of techniques designed to defuse impending violence or gain compliance via calming or directive touch. This can fail spectacularly if done incorrectly, so if you try it you will need to be prepared to jump to a higher level straightaway.

4. Empty-hand restraint—Use of techniques designed to control an aggressor through pain, or force compliance through leverage. This is what most martial sports focus on. The challenge is that a truly committed attacker won't be stopped by pain, and leverage cannot be applied indefinitely (especially if the other guy's got friends with him), so if this isn't working you will probably need to escalate. Also, if you do not have a duty to act you may be committing a crime by applying these techniques.

5. Less lethal force—Use of techniques or implements designed to incapacitate an aggressor while minimizing the likelihood of fatality or permanent injury. Many martial arts focus on this area, physiologically disabling the adversary's ability to continue fighting, which is a good thing since most street fights work at this level.

6. Lethal force—Use of techniques or implements likely to cause death or permanent injury. This often requires a weapon, though some techniques like chokes when misapplied or intentionally held too long will have the same result. Similarly, forcefully shoving (typically a lower level application) another person down a stairwell, onto a curb, or into the path of a moving vehicle can have lethal results; it's not just the application but also the environment in which you use it.

This scale of force should be applied sensibly to preserve your safety as the situation warrants. We've already said it, but it bears repeating: This is not like rungs of a ladder. You enter where you need to and jump around when necessary, rather than starting at the bottom and moving up if a particular level does not work.

There are no absolutes in self-defense, but your goal must be to apply sufficient force to effectively control the situation and keep yourself from harm without overdoing it. In general, you may legally use reasonable force in defending yourself. "Reasonable force" is considered only that force reasonably necessary to repel the attacker's force.

Exceeding a reasonable level of force may well turn a victim into a perpetrator in the eyes of the courts. Justifiable self-defense is a victim's defense to a criminal and/or civil charge. The legal reasoning goes like this: If your intent was to defend yourself then a reasonable person would only do so using reasonable force. Sounds a bit circular but it is very important. Using a higher level of force infers that you had intent to needlessly harm the other guy. This allows the perpetrator turned "victim" to use your defensive actions against you, the victim turned perpetrator. Even if a criminal prosecutor dismisses your actions, a civil court may not do so.

In other words, that means that if you overdo things, you're in trouble. Bad guys sue their victims all the time. They win too. It just isn't right, yet it happens in this litigious society. Clearly, if you underdo things, you'll lose the fight, which is trouble of a whole different kind. So, as Goldilocks learned in the fairytale, your response needs to be "just right."

Most confrontations can be resolved without violence. Even when it becomes necessary to go hands on, it is important to exercise a judicious level of force sufficient to control the other guy without overreacting.

Ethical Self-Defense

Bad things can happen whenever you fight, especially when you find yourself in a fight for your life. It's far better to avoid conflict and violence in the first place. Sometimes you see it coming and leave. Sometimes you can swallow your pride, apologize, and walk away. Sometimes you can capitulate, say handing your wallet to a mugger without a fight. But that doesn't mean that you shouldn't fight for everything you're worth if an encounter gets to the point where you have no other alternative but to do so (e.g., attempted rape or murder). Nevertheless, some folks feel that all countervailing force is morally wrong, that violence never solves anything. We strongly disagree.

The second paragraph of the Declaration of Independence proclaims, *"We hold these truths to be self-evident, that all men are created equal, that they are endowed by their Creator with certain unalienable Rights, that among these are Life, Liberty and the pursuit of Happiness."* Every person has a fundamental right to life, one that cannot be overridden by anyone save by the consequences of your own actions or by your own choosing. In other words, you have a fundamental right not to be killed. This right is a human entitlement, a mark of any civilized society.

But there is also a paramount reciprocity factor. It is possible to waive the right not to be killed by murdering or attempting to murder someone else. In other words, you have the duty not to kill or harm others so long as others adhere to the same duty toward you. It is the breakdown of this reciprocal relationship that explains why aggressors fail to have the right not to be killed by their victims, and why you possess the moral right to kill someone in self-defense if there is no other way to resolve a confrontation.

If someone makes an unprovoked attack against you, your friends, or your family, the aggressor is morally at fault for the attack and all consequences thereof. The defender is both morally and legally innocent so long as he or she acts within the true definition of self-defense, guarding him or herself against a real, imminent, and unavoidable threat of serious physical injury or death.

So, you have a fundamental right not to be killed, even if you must exercise countervailing force to safeguard that right. Further, you have a moral imperative to act in your own defense and possibly in the defense of others as well. As Edmund Burke so eloquently wrote, "All that is necessary for the triumph of evil is that good men do nothing." There are times when we are morally impelled to act. For some—law enforcement officers, soldiers, and security personnel to name a few—it is their job to run toward danger. For the rest of you, you must defend yourself if attacked directly and search your character in determining how to act if you come across an incident of violence toward someone else.

Justification

Fighting is illegal. And sometimes it's necessary. You already know that. Whenever you get into a fight, you face several risks, one of which is the possibility of having to justify your actions in court. You may know that too, but not what to do about it. Good people tend to make good decisions, but that doesn't necessarily mean that they explain them well enough to stay out of trouble, even with the benefit of expensive lawyers and expert witnesses to help out.

Here's the deal: It doesn't matter that you're the good guy if you fail to articulate it properly, oftentimes even when there's supporting video evidence. As stated earlier, self-defense is an affirmative plea, so it falls on you to explain. And the prosecutor will be doing his or her level best to trip you up every step along the way. You must be able to articulate exactly why you made each decision throughout the altercation. You can expect to be asked things like:

- Why did you get involved?
- Did you escalate an otherwise avoidable conflict?

- Why did you choose the level of force you selected?
- Why did you use the technique you used?
- What couldn't you have resolved this without hurting anyone?
- Why didn't you walk away?
- What the hell were you thinking?

Okay, maybe not that last one. But members of the jury are very likely wondering about that even if no one says it aloud. Prosecutors are adept at turning what seemed like a perfectly reasonable action at the time into something horrendous, selling it to the judge and jury, and obtaining a conviction. Their job is to win, and they're pretty good at it.

Here's another piece of bad news: If any martial arts training you have becomes public knowledge—not so hard in the YouTube/Facebook world today, not to mention a *dojo* or tournament website with your name on it—chances are good that it will be used against you in court. "Trained fighters" are typically held to a higher standard than everyday citizens (depending on jurisdiction) when it comes to prosecuting violence.

You can't just say that you were afraid for your life. That's talisman thinking and it never works. You need to be able to articulate exactly what the other guy did. How did you know that he had the intent, means, and opportunity to hurt you? And why couldn't you have simply walked away?

Easier said than done, right? But, you can practice.

Go to YouTube (or similar sites). Watch real fights. Oftentimes the altercation clearly led to a mutual fight despite the fact that both participants thought they were defending themselves. Pick a side. Was this person's actions legitimate self-defense? Look at all the times the guy who walked away could have been fine if only he had kept his mouth shut. Was the level of force used appropriate to the threat? Why?

There are times when pre-emptive strikes are justified and prudent, and others where such actions land the perpetrator in jail. Pretend you're in court and argue each guy's case. What were the pre-fight indicators that hinted at the danger? Was the level of force used reasonable? Why? It's easiest to see these things in retrospect, especially with a "replay" button, but once you get good at it, you will find it's not so hard to see the same things happening in "real life" up close and personal.

A Highly Selective Overview of Combative Arts throughout History

When we say selective history, we truly mean a selective history. It is virtually impossible to cover all of the combative arts across the globe in the range of human history, bind them together, and distribute them in a single volume. To that end, we made some choices based on accessibility, historical significance, touchstones, and representation.

There are, no doubt, unique combative arts that have never been recorded, or only moderately documented. Who knows what the hand-to-hand combat of the Mayan warrior looked like? Who knows what sort of hand-to-hand fighting the lost civilization that was swallowed by the Black Sea possessed? We can only piece together scraps of information that tell us the story; otherwise, these techniques are lost to time. Clearly, popularity and, in many instances, institutionalization preserved the historical hand-to-hand combat forms we know of today.

In some instances, the dogged determination and commitment of a few have preserved ancient fighting arts for us to see now. Even today, some hand-to-hand forms of sport are only regionally strong. An example might be collegiate wrestling in the United States. In 1972, Title IX was instituted at the collegiate level. Title IX required equal opportunities in funding for both men's and women's sports.

Because of the complications of funding, fan participation, and revenue generation, several sports that did not have large fan bases, high levels of participation, and (especially) revenue-generation were killed. Wrestling was one of those sports that suffered. Wrestling survives through the dedication and creativity of those committed to the sport, as well as lukewarm support by a parent institution. A case in point is the Pacific 12 conference, or "Pac-12," an athletic conference of twelve universities on the West Coast of the United States. Of these schools, only five, Arizona State, Oregon, Oregon State, Colorado, and Stanford, still muster wrestling teams.

Move your attention to the Midwest of America and you will see the Big 10, another athletic conference, and you will see on every university field a wrestling team. Wrestling is supported by the institutions, people, and athletes. An instance of this success is the University of Iowa, which has racked up 22 national championships.

Circumstances, geography, travel, communications, visionary individuals, and community support make all the difference in whether a person, a technique, or form of combat ever becomes more than just a local blip on the national or international radar screen.

We are convinced there were great grapplers and combatants who never made it into the annals of history. We are also fully aware that we are intentionally leaving out prominent and talented people whose accomplishments are well known. Some are left out due to numbers, niche arts, and artists aren't well known, and others because while they were brilliant at what they did, they were not necessarily adept at self-promotion. The greats who were lost to time may not have been the most pleasant people or possessed magnificent communication skills; they simply were extraordinary at combat.

A modern example of this might be the two ends of the spectrum when it comes to boxing: Heavyweight Champion Muhammad Ali was a remarkable communicator. Ali was loud, brash, singing his own praises in catchy rhymes and prose; he was tall, handsome, and tailor-made for the emerging modern marketing phenomenon of broadcast TV. On the other hand, you have Mike Tyson, a man whose life was wracked by trial and sadness. Both of these men, arguably the two most dominant personalities and boxers in the heavyweight division, are extremes at opposite ends of the spectrum. Yet it is intriguing to point out that quiet, efficient, and diligent Larry Holmes held the title of "Heavyweight Champion of the World" longer than any other man in modern history.

History is inconsistent, unfair, and oftentimes cruel. It can celebrate the notorious, exaggerate and grant powers and skills of legendary greatness to those undeserving of it.

The Battlefield

The battlefield of much of history involved hand-to-hand combat. Throwing a rock was a way to gain separation from an adversary while still striking him in an attempt to secure conquest. Throwing rocks begat using slings to gain more distance and more power because the farther you are from the other guy, the better the chance of your taking him out without getting hurt. Then spears and arrows became more deadly than the rocks. Soon shields and armor were developed to help blunt the impact of these weapons.

Skipping forward a bit, the use of gunpowder changed the level of engagement once again, sending what was effectively a rock faster, farther, and more accurately than any arrow. Then came high-tech armor to (somewhat) address the newfound velocities and projectiles. All of these were designed for stand-off positions where you could strike from relative safety. And then there's air power. The pilot who sees his adversary first wins. Like snipers, pilots know that if you see him before he sees you, you have an exceptionally high chance of killing him before he is even aware of your presence. Fail and you probably won't survive to learn the lesson.

The ground battle is similar in that if you can surprise the enemy, you have a high chance of success. Predatory animals operate in the same way. Watch any of the big cats: tigers, lions, cheetahs, or... well, not in person unless you're on safari with a big, honkin' rifle; TV's a lot safer. They all use stealth to close to striking distance unseen. The colors of their coats match the dry grass of the plains on which they hunt. They stay down wind so as not to have their scent give a clue to their prey that they are in the area. Crouching, moving slowly, all of these are tactics designed to gain the element of surprise. Once the predator is within striking distance, their prey is as good as dead. Striking distance is defined as the operational distance where a weapon can hit the target; for a cheetah this is the claws and jaws. The cat itself is the platform for its weapons.

This example of the big cats related to hand-to-hand combat is a good one because their methods are similar to hand-to-hand combat for humans. Cats want to make contact with the prey, bring it down, and then from a superior position destroy the prey's ability to survive. Mmm, meaty goodness…

The human battlefield is the same, be it in the desert, jungle, or city. Soldiers and civilians have different jobs, but in a predatory encounter, the tactics and results are pretty much the same. Unlike social violence where you're trying to gain status or prestige, predatory violence is putting the hurt on someone and/or taking their stuff. The street fighter knows he could be injured in a fair fight so he'll stack the deck against his victim, using weapons, ambushes, and other tactics that give him the advantage. Dialogue, distraction, and destruction are common. This means initiating contact with the enemy on your terms, obfuscating your intent, and kicking his ass. Keep a superior position, and kill (or rape or rob or assault or whatever) him.

To paraphrase Marc "Animal" MacYoung, "Him. Down. Now." We would add, "Insert weapon." Because you're the good guy, the choice of weapon could well be your fists or feet, but in a life or death struggle pretty much everything is on the table.

Pankration

> *"The pankratiasts, my boy, practice a dangerous brand of wrestling. They have to endure black eyes… and learn holds by which one who has fallen can still win, and they must be skillful in various ways of strangulation. They bend ankles and twist arms and throw punches and jump on their opponents."*
>
> —*Philostratos, On Gymnastics, second to third century* CE

Pankration was the ancient world's equivalent to modern Mixed Martial Arts. In 564 BCE, five hundred years before the birth of Christ, Arrichion of Phigalia a famous Olympian (*pankration* was an Olympic sport at that time) won a match while dead. His opponent whose name is lost to history had placed the Olympian in the "iron stranglehold," a hold which immobilized Arrichion. It is reported that Arrichion's trainer shouted to him the equivalent of, "What a fine funeral we will have if you don't submit." As legend goes, this cry from his trainer sparked Arrichion to make a drastic and serious play. In an attempt to weaken his opponent, Arrichion kicked at his opponent's feet, dislocating his adversary's right ankle. Some say Arrichion broke this opponent's foot, some say he dislocated toes. Nonetheless, damage was done. Arrichion, who was a finalist for a third consecutive time in the Olympics, was not going to let victory slip away.

After the foot attack, Arrichion pitched his body to the left in an effort to wrest his neck clear of the iron stranglehold. The opponent found the move too painful to bear and immediately signaled, submitting to Arrichion. The opponent released Arrichion only to find the lifeless body of the Olympian on top of him, dead of a broken neck. When Arrichion had tossed his body to the left in an attempt to escape, he snapped his own neck in much the same way a hangman's noose snaps a condemned man's neck. Nevertheless, Arrichion was declared the winner of the match because his opponent had submitted. To a dead man.

Pankration as Olympic Sport

Pankration is a form of sport and combat that combines wrestling and boxing. It had been in practice prior to its introduction to the Olympic Games in 648 BCE. *Pankration* did not replace wrestling or boxing as an Olympic sport; it was an entirely different competition.

Greek mythology holds that Hercules and Theseus created *pankration* while battling opponents such as the Minotaur of the Labyrinth and the first labor of Hercules, the Nemean Lion, whose pelt Hercules is often portrayed wearing. In competition, knockouts were common and many of the matches went to the ground where striking, strangulation, joint locks, and/or dislocations were used to either make the opponent unconscious or submit. Approximately four hundred years after the death of Christ, the Romans incorporated *pankration* into their entertainment, right alongside the gladiatorial battles. If a participant did break one of the few rules that governed the match, biting or eye-gouging, the referee enforced the rules with a large stick, mercilessly beating the cheater.

The match would begin from a standing position, so opening techniques were designed to bridge the distance between the two competitors. Kicks and punches served that need. As the fighters grew closer, elbows and knees became the preferred weapons. This type of fighting might remind you of western boxing or *muay Thai*. However, with little restriction on techniques you would see strikes banned in western boxing such as a backfist or a hammerfist. One way to look at the hand techniques of *pankration* is this way: everything was legal. You could strike with any part of your hand: the palm, the forefist, or the sides. Target-wise, other than eye strikes everything else was fair game, even rabbit punches, downward elbow strikes to the neck, and other hazardous applications that are banned in modern competitions.

The *pankration* kicks were low, focusing on the stomach, groin and legs, and included sweeps. The *gastrizein* is the signature front kick of *pankration*. The prefix *gastro* is Greek in origin, and means stomach. The target of the *gastrizein* is clearly in the name, the stomach. The *gastrizein* used the heel of the kicking foot in combination with a thrusting strike that was immediately followed by a shoving motion with the leg. This kick is built around the lever action of the heel, knee and hip, all working in concert with the thigh muscle. It was a truly powerful weapon.

If you have not had an opportunity to see, or worse feel the *gastrizein*, you can see it in the hyper-stylized movie *300*, directed by Zack Snyder, and which was based on the graphic novel of the same name by Frank Miller. In a scene early in the movie, King Xerxes has sent a messenger to Sparta to tell them to surrender. King Leonidas, having none of this, yells out the now famous line, "This is Sparta!" and uses the *gastrizein* to kick Xerxes' messenger into a well.

An interesting aspect of the competition was a method to end a match that had gone on too long. The method was called a *klimax*, which translates into "ladder," implying the top of the ladder, or the final rung. The fighters were separated and a coin toss was made. The winner was allowed to strike first, unopposed. This was somewhat similar to a pistol duel. If the punch was successful, the deliverer won, but if the opponent didn't fall he was proclaimed the winner and advanced to the next round.

Pankration in Combat

As a training tool for combat, *pankration* knew no master. Used by the Greek soldiers and Spartan Hoplites, *pankration* training and techniques were also used by Alexander the Great's phalanxes as they engaged in hand-to-hand combat. The techniques and strategies employed in *pankration* clearly worked, and worked well. Eventually the entire Greek military and all of the various city-states employed *pankration* in their hand-to-hand training.

An example of a technique used in *pankration* that might seem unusual to a grappler today might be the trachea grab. The technique is simple in that the attacker reaches out and literally grabs the opponent's throat—the trachea, or windpipe—with a claw-like hand, squeezing the opponent's throat in the clutch. Although this technique was used in combat, it was also used in the sport end of the art. Such competitions, as you might imagine, were brutal.

Banning Pankration

Theodosius I, the last emperor of a unified Roman empire, eventually banned *pankration* in 393 CE. This edict was issued at the same time he banned the gladiatorial contests and all pagan festivals in order to wipe the empire clean of things that were considered counter to the Christian ethos. By this time, *pankration* had been part of the gladiatorial games for quite a while and, therefore, it was lumped in with the ban. This effectively put an end to institutional *pankration*; however, it continued to survive in small pockets and regions where the decree from the emperor was not pronounced or just outright ignored.

Modern Pankration

Many dedicated modern organizations and individuals are making great efforts to keep *pankration* alive. Some would argue that the modern MMA movement is a rebirth of *pankration*, while others will say that MMA is not *pankration*, or a watered-down version of the art. We're not going to weigh in on that argument, but we will state that there is a lot to be learned from this no-holds barred fighting style. What you train is more or less what you will do under duress, albeit to a lesser degree of ability due to adrenaline and whatnot. Clearly pankratiasts understood and trained for this.

Mongolian Wrestling, Bökh

Mongolian wrestling, or *bökh*, is one of the older, continuously practiced forms of wrestling in the world. It reaches back to the time of the great Genghis Khan (1162–1227 CE), the Mongolian warrior chieftain who united the nomadic tribes of Northeast Asia. Khan used wrestling to help keep his military in shape for battle. There are different versions of Mongolian wrestling with slightly different rules. However, the basics are the same throughout the regions: Make your opponents touch their upper body or elbow to the ground. In more severe versions of Mongolian wrestling, it begins to look like Japanese *sumo* in that no other body part may touch the ground other than the soles of the feet.

One of the most significant aspects of Mongolian wrestling is that there are no weight classes. This is unusual in sports. The reason is that *bökh* has retained the battlefield combative aspect of the art's origin. The refusal to segregate competitors by weight class is reflective of the battlefield. In combat, mismatches of size and weight are actively sought. After all, the larger fighter is always seeking the smaller opponent in an effort to achieve victory as swiftly as possible. Let's face it, the more mass you bring to the battle and the greater the mismatch, the lower the likelihood of your being injured. Furthermore, you expend less energy.

Bökh still honors this fundamental aspect of battle and retains this mismatch to make the weaker fighter stronger through technique, intelligence, and experience. Since the same thing happens in predatory attacks on the street, where virtually all women and most men are outmatched in size and strength by their attackers, there is a lot to be learned here.

Bökh as a Sport

Naadam, or "play," is the name of the festival that takes place in July and August throughout Mongolia. Matches require no special ring or mat and are done in an open grassy field. While most forms of competition use lottery and brackets to arrange the matches, *bökh* is different. The host of the festival has the absolute and unquestioned authority to set the pairings. This schema was not at all just, intentionally so, and often visiting wrestlers were given poor opportunities to advance while local wrestlers were favored. The modern bracket method, in use since 1980, is considered a more equitable distribution of talent and weights, although it still retains the tradition of mismatched pairings.

Bökh wrestlers are ranked, with ranks proceeding, from the list below, from highest to lowest (the higher the number the higher the level). Wrestlers are also ranked by rounds, so several wrestlers will carry the same title, or level:

- Champion–Titan
- 9th–Lion
- 8th–Garuda
- 7th–Elephant
- 6th–Hawk
- 5th–Bird

Bökh in Combat

The rules and the attitude that was propagated by this sport could clearly be taken to the battlefield with little adjustment. As we know, one of the worst things that could happen on a battlefield to you would be to lose your footing and find yourself on the ground. You can lose your footing by your own accord or be thrown to the ground by an enemy combatant. Regardless, you're on the ground, a horrible place to be in a fight. Whether it's in the mud and blood of ancient battlefield or garbage strewn alley amongst discarded condoms and used needles, it's damnably hard to fight without mobility.

The Mongolian wrestling rules state that putting your free hand, your knee(s), or your shoulder on the ground means you lose the match. These rules grew out of the knowledge that if you have one palm on the ground you now have only one hand with which to fight. On the battlefield, this translates into being put in a position of fighting upward toward the enemy in a defensive encounter with one side of your body.

In most battlefield cases, you will not have to fight long from this position because you will be killed; the other guy's got weapons after all. As stated earlier, the competition is held outside on a grassy field, not on an indoor facility or a modern mat. This outdoor and natural environment is a direct link to the anticipated battlefield. Although a flat field with consistent terrain is sought, little can be done in preparation for bumps in the ground, rocks, and slippery footing on the grass. As the day wears on, the field becomes torn up, grass and dirt mixing together, making for uneven and spotty footing.

Indian Wrestling, Kushti

Many forms of Indian wrestling have existed over the thousands of years that the culture has been around. Over that time, travelers between cultures in the proximity to India, and even those far away, have been exposed to Indian wrestling. In fact, Bodhidharma is rumored to have brought martial arts from India to the Shaolin temple in China where they later spread across the sea to Okinawa, Japan, Korea, and much of the rest of the world. The sheer size of India had resulted in regional derivations of wrestling, often integrating the whims of local ideas of competition. These differences and variations are difficult to categorize. *Kushti*, once limited to royalty in India, is nowadays considered the national sport of that country.

Traditional *kushti* was done in earthen pits that were prepared with a blend of clay and soil to create a uniform, flat fighting surface. Further, the Indian wrestlers lived together in stables much like their brethren, the Japanese *sumo* wrestlers. Continuing the analogy, strict rules outlined their daily life, including what they could eat and how they were allowed to use their free time. The use of alcohol and tobacco were forbidden. Wrestlers also abstained from carnal relations. Clearly, the art of *kushti* represented a way of life and not just an athletic diversion.

The wrestlers' diet was unique. Dominated by milk, *ghee* (clarified butter), and almonds, their diet was designed to aid in strength and stamina. Fruits and vegetables were also incorporated to bring balance to the meals. The training was done in a stable-like atmosphere under the direction of a *guru*, a recognized expert. In the West, we associate this term with a spiritual leader, which it can be, yet it is also used in other aspects of life. A *kushti guru* was a teacher with great knowledge and experience.

The training hall or gymnasium was called an *akharas*. It was filled with supplemental training aids designed to strengthen the wrestlers who toiled there. These classic training aids included clubs that could look like bowling pins (*joris*), as well as barbells (*sumtola*), stone weights (*nals*), and other implements. Similar to *hojo undo* in classical Japanese martial arts, these methods of strengthening the wrestlers' bodies used any available resource in order to gain an edge over opponents. This edge in strength and stamina was honed for maximum benefit. Such things are universal in the martial arts world, as old as the oldest art.

Like many other forms of wrestling, the rules of *kushti* are simple: throw your opponent to the ground so that he lands on his back. Choke holds and armbars are also used to make an opponent submit. Controlling an adversary and using pain compliance to make him submit are time honored wrestling fundamentals, but you don't need to dedicate your life to an art form in order to make use of them in the ring or on the street.

Burns, Gotch, and Hackenschmidt

Farmer Burns (1861–1937), Frank Gotch (1878–1917), and George Hackenschmidt (1878–1968) were three men who dominated the world of catch-as-catch-can wrestling. Prominent in American wrestling during the early 1900s, all were born within a seventeen-year period, and all knew and competed with each other. These three men took advantage of the modern press and brought "catch wrestling" to the public eye, making it a major attraction.

Some might say that putting these three men into one measly chapter sells them short, reducing each man into a shadowed outline, doing a disservice to all three. Yup, we agree. But, as stated previously, this is a martial arts manual, not a history book. Yeah, these three men were giants who had significant impacts not only on their art, but also on modern day sports; however, we will just touch on some of the key points of their lives for our purposes.

Traditionally catch wrestling did not include striking. As the name implies, it was about attacking your opponent where he was, making use of what was given to you. This might mean reaching out and grabbing the opponents lead arm, because that was the easiest thing available. Then, exploiting the initial point of contact, wherever you caught a hold of your opponent, you gained control and caused him to submit. In this example, it might mean pulling the opponent's lead arm, working an elbow lock, and driving him to the ground.

The oldest of these men was Farmer Burns. His given first name was Martin. Born in Iowa in 1861, Martin's father died when he was eleven years old, so he had to begin working early in life. It fell to Martin to support his mother, brother, and five sisters by toiling at a nearby farm. The situation sucked to be sure, but all this hard work turned him into an exceptionally strong individual at a very young age. With a demonstrated flair for wrestling, he entered his first match at age nineteen.

His match against wrestler David Graft was declared a draw after two hours and nineteen minutes, remarkable considering modern competitions. Martin soon dropped his first name in favor of the moniker "Farmer," a nod to his Iowan agrarian roots. Farmer Burns weighed in at about one-hundred and sixty-five pounds, yet boasted a twenty-inch neck that he developed after a losing match with Henry Clayton. Using full nelsons, (illegal in modern amateur wrestling), chicken wings, and creative pinning combinations, Farmer Burns built an impressive winning record.

Farmer Burns' greatest contribution was his methods of training and his coaching. This legacy led to the University of Iowa becoming a perennial powerhouse in college wrestling. It was also the basis for some highly advertised modern strength and conditioning systems.

While still wrestling in the catch-as-catch-can circuit, Farmer Burns met and bested a young man named Frank Gotch, another Iowan. After losing to Burns at the age of twenty-one, Gotch joined him as his prized student, benefiting from Burns' excellent teaching methods. Soon Gotch was on his way. He wrestled all comers regardless of age or size. His travels took him as far as the mining camps of Alaska, remote towns in Canada, and all across the Midwest. In Chicago, he defeated "The Russian Lion," George Hackenschmidt, to earn the world title in 1908. Gotch continued to barnstorm for several years and retired after breaking his leg in a match. He died in 1917 at thirty-nine years of age.

George Hackenschmidt, born in Estonia in 1878, was nicknamed the Russian Lion. A bodybuilder and wrestler, he was only twenty-three years old when he defeated Ahmed Madrali, winning the European Championship in 1901. Reported to have had some two thousand wrestling matches, he suffered only five losses. Hackenschmidt was the creator of the popular weight lifting exercise the "Hack Squat" as well as being an advocate of weighted workouts. It is also reported that Hackenschmidt was injured in a training session a few days prior to his match with Gotch, hence not in top form for the 1908 competition at Cominsky Park.

Modern catch-as-catch-can wrestlers such as Stu Hart from Calgary (1915–2003), the father of professional wrestlers Bret "The Hitman" Hart and Owen Hart, transitioned from the barnstorming time of Burns, Hackenschmidt, and Gotch to modern television where professional wrestling gained massive popularity. For insight into Stu Hart and his family, we recommend the documentary about Bret Hart titled *Wrestling with Shadows*. You will get a chance to see and hear some of the lifestyle, as well as the practice and discipline that goes into the life of a catch-as-catch-can wrestler.

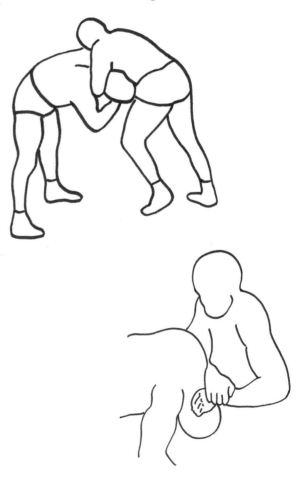

Examples of the modern wrestlers of the catch-as-catch-can world are Erik Paulson, Frank Shamrock, Ken Shamrock, and many others. These men might well be considered mixed martial artists because they are just as adept at using a submission to secure victory as their fists and feet. They might have competed in a "show," but they were accomplished martial artists in the true sense of the word.

To demonstrate the subtlety between sport and combat, look at this picture of George Hackenschmidt with his assistants. The techniques used by these wrestlers bordered on the ability to maim, or seriously injure, an opponent at almost every turn. These pictures are from Hackenschmidt's book, *The Complete Science of Wrestling*, first published in 1909.

This is noted as being a fair hold. Nevertheless, a subtle shifting of the dominant wrestler's arms will result in the mouth and nose of the other man becoming covered, leading to his suffocation. Without clearing the face to get air, the man will quickly pass out, leaving him defenseless. This hold is not that big a deal in the ring with oversight by referees and medical professionals, but it sucks blocky nuts on the street. Hell, any strangulation technique done improperly or held too long can kill.

A front chancery and bar hold can also become exceptionally dangerous by wrenching the neck and moving the dominant wrestler's right hand to a shoulder, resulting in a spraining of the neck and a tearing of the shoulder. This not only hurts like hell, but it can also render the shoulder, and subsequently the arm, useless for further combat.

Jack Dempsey, Boxer

There are a great many great boxers out there, but we want to focus on Jack Dempsey because not only was he an extraordinary competitor, he was also a fighter who served to transition boxing into the modern age. Jack Dempsey (1895–1983) was born in Manassa, Colorado, and began fighting at an early age. Leaving his family at age sixteen, he traveled the West, fighting to make a living. He turned professional and began to amass an impressive record.

In 83 fights, he had 66 wins (51 via knockout), 6 losses, and 11 draws. To put this in perspective, look at his percentages: Dempsey won 80% of his fights, 77% by knockout. To further illustrate the significance of this record, compare it to now-retired champion Joe Calzaghe, who retired undefeated with a record of 46 and 0, never losing a professional fight, and held the WBO super middleweight title for a decade. Clearly these fighters are from different time periods, but let's run the numbers anyway. Dempsey fought 82 fights, while Calzaghe had 46. Dempsey fought 46% more fights than Calzaghe and Dempsey knocked out more fighters by about 9%. These are impressive records for both men and no disrespect for their accomplishments is intended.

Dempsey was a mauler and a brawler, not an Olympic-style point boxer. Dempsey made this famous quote that typifies his attitude about boxing and fighting: "You're in there for three-minute rounds with gloves on and a referee. That's not real fighting."

Dempsey went on to write books and train the U.S. military. The most significant book he wrote was the classic *Championship Fighting: Explosive Punching and Aggressive Defense*, first published in 1950. This book breaks down Dempsey's philosophies of leverage, punching, bobbing, and weaving. We strongly recommend that the reader seek a copy of Dempsey's book because it demonstrates knowledge honed not only in boxing rings, but also in the bars throughout the West and Midwest. We believe that the secret of Dempsey's techniques can be found in the subtitle, *Aggressive Defense*.

Dempsey shows you his understanding of defense, important to any sport, but vital in street fighting where losing cannot be an option. For those who practice karate, you will be amazed at how similar his style is to the classical Okinawan and Japanese arts in terms of body alignment and power generation. In fact, we showed his book to an Okinawan karate expert. He could not read the English, but upon looking at the illustrations exclaimed, "This guy is a *karateka*!" He wasn't, but Dempsey was far more than just a boxer.

Jujitsu

Japanese *jujitsu* is a form of hand-to-hand combat originating in feudal Japan. The brutal takedowns, locks, throws, chokes, pins, and other moves were developed for battle-field combat by the *samurai* who needed to be able to fight in any circumstances, even if temporarily disarmed.

The word, *ju* in Japanese means "soft." To that point, the techniques of *jujitsu* were designed and implemented using leverage, imbalance, and, in many instances, the opponent's momentum to make applications work. *Jujitsu* was not standardized during its establishment because there were many different sword systems that incorporated hand-to-hand combat in their training. Nevertheless, the core principles of *jujitsu* generally remained uniform even where the techniques varied because of this dispersed development. After all, there are a limited number of vital areas that can be attacked and only so many ways that various portions of the body can be manipulated.

There is no one way that *jujitsu* became popular; it began to enter into the general public through various venues. *Samurai* who no longer had employment after the Meiji Restoration often had no discernible skills other than the art of warfare. Consequently, these out-of-work warriors often began teaching the hand-to-hand aspects of their art to earn a living.

Like other martial arts, the techniques of *jujitsu* were designed to take advantage of the weaknesses of the human body, but unlike other styles they were also designed to work on an armored opponent. In general, hand strikes, such as a closed-fist karate punch, proved to be ineffective against armored adversaries. Attacking joints such as the elbow or knee, on the other hand, exploited the seams in the armor. Further, throwing the opponent to the ground placed the enemy in an inferior position, severely compromising his ability to fight, let alone defend himself against armed and armored adversaries. If you could do it simultaneously while dislocating a joint or causing blunt force trauma to the head or neck so much the better.

Even for unarmored adversaries it was a useful skill. At one time, *jujitsu* schools across Japan numbered in the thousands.

Judo

The name judo translates from Japanese meaning "the gentle way." An Olympic sport, judo is taught in schools and universities across the globe today.

Originating in Japan, judo was developed from *jujitsu* by Professor Jigoro Kano in 1882. Kano removed the most dangerous techniques from the *jujitsu* syllabus over time. Examples of banned techniques include leg and ankle locks. After the dangerous techniques were banned, it became safer to participate. The combat art was transformed into a sport. A victory in a judo tournament can be secured by throwing the opponent to the ground so that he lands on his back. Other means of winning are submission, via pinning, arm lock, or choke. You can also earn more points than your opponent.

A *gi* (uniform) is worn by each participant. The *gi* is required be of certain lengths, such as the sleeves and pant legs, to insure fair and equal access to grips. In the past, judo competitors were identified by red and white cloths tied around the waist. In modern competition, the fighters wear contrasting uniforms, one blue and the other white. The traditional judo *gi* is made of an extra-heavy weave to withstand the strain because it is used as a key component for executing techniques.

Many strong competitors and innovators are significant in the history of judo. The following is a brief, and, therefore, incomplete list of some of these *judoka*:

1. Jigoro Kano: The founder of judo, educator and teacher.
2. Kyuzo Mifune: Considered one of the greatest technical practitioners of judo.
3. Masahiko Kimura: A 5th degree black belt by age 18, he was one of the greatest proponents of arm locks.
4. Trevor Leggett: The author of some 30 books regarding judo.
5. Nobuyuki Sato: A two-time world champion and former head coach of the Japanese national team.
6. Yasuhiro Yamashita: The most successful *judoka* of the modern age, he has won five gold medals in world competition and 203 consecutive victories.

Of interest, *Sanshiro Sugata*, the first movie by famed director Akira Kurosawa, was the story of a man who set out to learn *jujitsu* and convert it into judo. Sounds kinda familiar, huh?

While modern judo is a sport, the traditional syllabus includes striking techniques, disarms, and a host of street-worthy applications. With little modification, judo techniques can be used for self-defense, particularly against adversaries who do not know how to fall correctly.

When you get to the techniques section, you will undoubtedly note that we use judo terminology quite a bit when describing applications. This is not intended as a show of favoritism. These techniques are common to virtually every grappling art and many striking arts as well; we simply chose commonly understood language for clarity, which is sort of amusing—using Japanese nomenclature to ensure that English speakers know what we're talking about—but it is a testament to how widespread judo truly has become.

Samozashchita Bez Oruzhiya (Sambo)

Samozashchita bez oruzhiya, or *sambo*, is a Russian style of hand-to-hand combat developed initially by and for the Russian military. The name of the art translates to "self-defense without weapons." It was developed in the 1920s by several individuals, Viktor Oshchecpkov, Viktor Spiridonov, and Spiridonov's student Anatoly Kharalampiev.

Viktor Oshchecpkov spent several years in Japan, training intermittently at the Kodokan from 1911 to 1917. He eventually earned a 2nd degree black belt in judo. It is important to know that at that time judo had only five degrees of black belt, so this was a more impressive accomplishment than it might seem today. The Bolshevik Revolution, or October Revolution, led by Vladimir Lenin spread across Russia in the fall of 1917, ending Oshchecpkov's travels to Japan. Sadly, Oshchecpkov was executed by order of Joseph Stalin, Lenin's successor, in 1937.

In 1918, Lenin ordered and established *vseobuch*, an abbreviation for "general military training," which would serve as the breeding ground for the development of *sambo*. In the 1920s, Oshchecpkov's work in hand-to-hand combat was merged with other systems with the intent to develop a combative system for the Red Army. Into this union went everything that had combative value, drawing from various sources such as Mongolian, Georgian, Romanian, and other wrestling systems. Many regional forms of combat were pulled into the system. While it may have more or less originated with judo, the development of *sambo* was closed off to the rest of the world due to Communist restrictions on travel, communication, and commerce. This gave *sambo* a distinctive and focused environment within which to develop in unique ways.

Viktor Spiridonov suffered war injuries during World War I. Because of those injuries, he had to grapple in a different manner, a way that required less power and more leverage and subtlety. It is said that his style had a softer edge, similar to the Japanese art of *aikido*.

Anatoly Kharalampiev is called the father of *sambo*, as he used his connections within the political system and maneuvered to get the USSR Committee of Sports to adopt *sambo* as the official combat sport in 1938. This gave *sambo* an official year of birth, something lacking in so many combative sports' due to their organic evolution.

Competitors are broken down into weight divisions as well as gender and age. Similar to western wrestling, victory can be secured by submission, or points, ranging from 1, 2, and 3, depending on the throw and the result. Unlike judo, however, there is no victory by a single throw in *sambo*.

Dry Fire (or How to Get Good Faster, Better, and if not Cheaper at least More Effectively)

In 1886, the police department of the Tokyo Metropolitan Police held a contest to determine what school would teach the Tokyo police officers martial arts. The concept was straightforward; the best school would win because, as logic would have it, they possessed the best techniques and training methods. Then the police would learn from the victorious school.

The Kodokan judo club made it to the mat for the competition, and the results were significant. Out of nine matches between the *jujitsu* school and the fledgling judo club, the Kodokan won eight of the matches. With no time limits on a match, the final match between Saigo and Terujima lasted some fifteen minutes, finally ending with Terujima being thrown so hard that he suffered a concussion.

Kodokan judo won the contract to train the Tokyo Metropolitan Police, helping put judo on the fast track to becoming the world-wide sport that it is today.

While both judo and *jujitsu* had the same origins, the methods, not the techniques, made the difference between victory and defeat. Having said that, before we can discuss the methods that separated these fighters and systems, we first need to address the techniques. Kano removed many of the techniques that had high injury rates from the judo canon. When two fighters matched up for the competition, the *judoka* never looked at the legs as an option in the same light as a the *jujitsuka*. The *jujitsu* practitioners, on the other hand, had the option of attacking the legs, knees, and ankles. The question then is, why, with all of these extra items available, did the *jujitsu* team lose eight out of nine fights?

Initially, it makes sense that having more techniques in a system would give the contestants a consistent and profound edge. Further, the length of time the *jujitsu* school was in existence was vastly longer than the upstart judo club. These facts could lead one to believe that with the combination of these two advantages, more techniques and more experience, the *jujitsu* practitioners would handily defeat the *judoka*.

If we had been present for this competition, we would have bet all the money in our pockets that *jujitsu* would win and do so decisively. Wouldn't you? So what was the "magic bullet" that secured victory? We submit to you that it is the concept of "dry fire."

Dry fire is a term used to describe the practice of aiming a firearm at a target and pulling the trigger without a bullet in the chamber. Sounds simple, but it isn't really. The idea is that you get a chance to practice the act of preparing to use your weapon, your technique, in a slow, controlled process much like *kata* (forms practice). Proper stance, arm motion, handgrip, sight picture, and trigger press are all perfected without worrying about recoil. Whether you are planning to use a firearm or practice a hand-to-hand technique, working the fundamentals in a controlled environment has a profound impact on how you will perform "live," when the shit hits the fan.

For those of you that have judo experience, this might be equated to the training process of *uchi komi*, the repetitive and swift action of stepping into a technique, not throwing, and getting back out of the technique ready to repeat. The key to *uchi komi* is the proper position and proper technique. This practice makes entries during a tournament stronger, faster, and far more likely to yield success.

The idea for dry fire for a gun carries with it some simple practices, which are also clearly applicable to hand-to-hand sport or unarmed combat. Here are some key points for getting the most value from such practice:

- Dry fire often, and with regularity. This is one of those "no shit" things. Giving a mini lecture on the benefits of frequent and regular practice to the reader would be condescending at this point, so let us move on.

- Know the key points of the motion you are practicing. The key points are actually three places, the beginning, the middle, and the end. However, the beginning position and the final position are paramount. If you start strong and end strong, the intervening motion is invariably correct. Get into position to begin your repetitions. If the beginning of a movement is correct and the final position is correct, then the middle point pretty much takes care of itself.

- Go slow. Going slow at the outset of the movement allows for analysis. An analysis is just that, an opportunity to look at it and understand what you are doing. This is the phase where a pattern, a union of mind and technique, can begin to establish itself. This "muscle memory" helps assure that you will perform well under duress.

- Use training aids. With a handgun, many practitioners place a small coin or a marble on top so that if they jerk the trigger or make any sudden, rough movements, it will fall off. Similarly, using mirrors or filming your practice can help point out subconscious flaws in your technique. Feedback from partners and observant practitioners helps too.

- Finally, go at speed. When you do it for real, all the practice time spent in dry fire comes into play. You can see the benefits of the training. In the judo example, your entries become swift and powerful. The execution of your technique is compelling, the completion final and definitive.

This practice method accelerates a practitioner's mastery of the art, most any fighting art. It also helps you understand modifications that might be necessary depending on whether you are working to a sport, drunkle, or combative application. For example, while throws are very effective in all three scenarios, you can't just walk up and slap one on an adversary in the street. There's no grip and jockeying for position as you would find in a sporting match. Consequently a "blow before throw" modification must be made to set up the technique. Hit the guy, and then execute the throw before he recovers enough to defend himself. You get the idea.

Entry

An entry in the martial arts can best be referred to as crossing from your personal space into your opponent's personal space, or, conversely, them entering into your space. This entry is designed to gain advantage over the opponent and dominate them. If you can enter strongly enough, victory is almost a foregone conclusion.

Here are some basic entries that a person can use: the Boxer, the Wrestler, and the Daylight Dracula, each described in detail below. There are other means of entry and they can vary in body, hand, and foot positions as well as angles, resulting in many versions of these three basic forms. Different forms of combat require different forms of entry. Some are designed around sport rules, while others are designed around combative situations.

Simply put, form follows the function of the environment. The Boxer will enter with a fist, striking the opponent and following up with a flurry of punches when and as the openings appear. The Wrestler will enter via a grab, hook, or scoop, using these techniques to ground the adversary and gain the submission he seeks. The Daylight Dracula blends these two coming from its originating art *jujitsu* and allows the participant to do whatever works without restrictions.

There are others, of course, such as the SPEAR™ (Spontaneous Protection Enabling Accelerated Response), but we're only going to cover these three as they are solid representations of three different strategies. These beginning entry positions should not be judged on their content, but on their context. The Daylight Dracula could be weak and susceptible to the single or double leg take down the Wrestler might provide, whereas the Boxer might have trouble with the Daylight Dracula. You can quickly see that these matchups are similar to the classic rock-paper-scissors game.

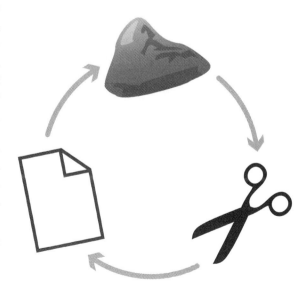

Rock smashes scissors, scissors cut paper, and paper smashes rock; as with everything in martial arts, each has its own strengths and weaknesses.

The Boxer

There are many different kinds of boxing stances; however, the key elements of a boxing style, the feet are positioned slightly wider than the shoulders to create a good base. The stance should not be so wide as to sacrifice mobility, however. Three classic positions are the upright, the semi-crouch, and the full crouch. The upright position can best be described as the old bare knuckles stance used by such fighters as John L. Sullivan. The

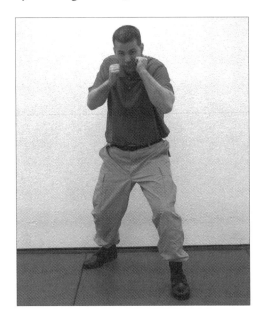

more modern semi-crouch is oftentimes seen in Olympic boxing whereas the full-crouch was employed famously by former Olympic and World Heavyweight champion Smokin' Joe Frazer.

The closed fists up around the head are a feature of the modern boxing stance. This hand position allows the head to be protected from incoming strikes. Hits below the belt are illegal in boxing, and body blows require significant repetition to cause injury to a well-conditioned athlete, so the fastest way to end a boxing match is to shut his brain down by hitting him in the head until you get a knockout. To do that, you need to hit the head with enough force to cause a neurological knockout (and, frequently, a concussion).

The boxer has a simple goal; hit the other guy in the head until he falls down. His stances help him slip past the other guy's defensive position to land his blows. Stand-up fighters on the street often use similar techniques. Spend a little time on YouTube.com watching actual brawls and you'll see what we mean.

The Wrestler

The wrestler's beginning stance is designed to move forward in an explosive manner, yet it is balanced to be able to simultaneously defend against an explosive forward assault from the other guy. To achieve this twofold goal, the wrestler usually adopts a stance wider than what a boxer would use. The knees of the wrestler are bent more deeply than a boxer's too. His hands are open, held around the chest area so that he can reach out and grab. This hand position also serves as a means of defense against an opponent's grab or shoot. By "shoot" we are referring to the single- or double-leg takedown where a wrestler grabs one or both of his adversary's legs and drives forward to bring the other guy to the ground. This beginning position allows for a wide variety of entries, techniques that can be executed on both the vertical and the horizontal line.

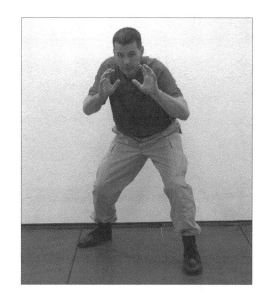

Once again, this style is not limited to the ring. There are a lot of grapplers out there, many of whom get into street fights or barroom brawls from time to time. Assuming an escalation between the initial conflict and the fight, it may be possible to judge whether or not the other guy has martial arts training as well as his preferred attack methodology simply by the stance he adopts and the way in which he breathes and moves. Low, slow breathing and smooth gait are pretty good indicators of a skilled adversary.

Daylight Dracula (or Hiji Ate)

The Daylight Dracula can be found on the street, in classical arts such as *jujitsu* and some karate systems, or in pretty much any workshop conducted by Rory Miller, who coined the term. The idea behind the Daylight Dracula is to guard your face and throat while charging the opponent. It's a great counterambush technique, one that allows you to react to an attack in a manner that takes initiative away from the other guy, even if you're behind in the count (bad pun intended).

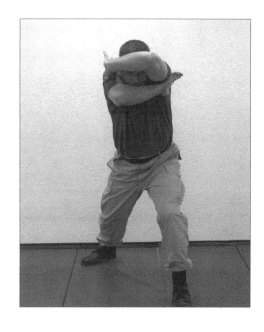

The offensive concept behind Daylight Dracula is to close the distance, invade the opponent's space, and place him on his heels. Placing the opponent on his heels, as we know, makes it difficult to retaliate without righting oneself and regaining balance. The combination of parry/block along with the strike makes this technique a powerful and effective entry. The bladed "archer" stance provides forward momentum while reducing your target area in a way that can help blows slide off.

Clearly, there are other methods of accomplishing the same thing, such as SPEAR™. It's the principle that counts, not the technique.

Macto Bicallis

Macto bicallis is pronounced "maw toe buy callis." A Latin term that, loosely translated, it means "the fighting way." To simply call it that, however, is not doing the Latin roots of the words justice. *Macto* can be translated to mean several things besides fighting, including magnify, glorify, honor, slay, punish, or afflict. The word *bicallis* means footpath. So you can see that the possible definitions can range from "the glory path" to "the walk of honor," or even "the path of punishment."

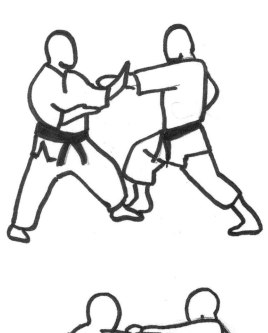

The *macto bicallis* is a powerful training aid that can help you explore tactical options and ultimately aid in discovering your fighting tendencies. It is a form of clinical study of your body that helps you build on your natural inclinations such that what you do under duress works in concert with your proclivities rather than against them. You guessed it. That tends to end well, even when adrenalized.

Often in classical schools of martial arts, a standard application (*bunkai oyo* in Japanese) is applied to any given martial movement. This is the accepted interpretation of your interaction with an opponent. An example of this would be the common application of side stepping to the outside of an incoming punch, blocking the punch in some manner, and returning a counterstrike. Another version of this would be to step to the inside, opening the opponent, blocking, and reposting.

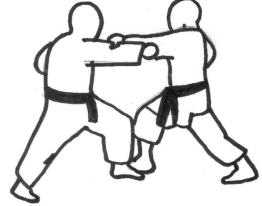

In essence, these two responses are the same thing. If you perform the response solo, as when performing a *kata* or form, the motions appear identical.

So, these two responses are really the same thing done differently.

Fighting, whether on the street or in the ring, doesn't have to be complicated. The ability to do a handful of techniques extremely well is a pathway to success. However, the study of other options can assist you in becoming a smarter fighter. Sometimes it's using more complex techniques, while other times it's doing simple stuff with unusual angles. The more experience you have, the more apparent it will be when something is not working and the easier it will be to seamlessly shift to a secondary application. In police training, this can often be seen in training exercises where the rookie officers are placed into situations by their trainers, scenarios that are designed to make the rookie's

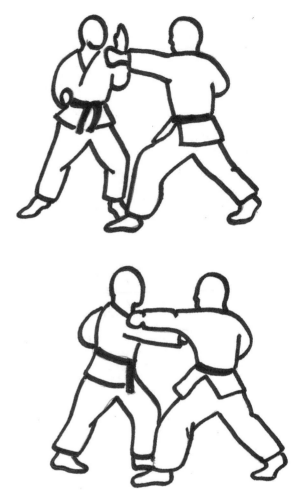

preferred technique fail. If nothing else, this broadens the trainee's thought process which in the training hall is far more important than merely learning new techniques.

Not everything discovered during this type of training will ever be applied. And some things not intended may ultimately prove to be of great benefit. Take a non-martial arts example: you may have heard of Post-it Notes®. You know, those ubiquitous paper squares with a little bit of adhesive attached to the backside we use for… well, almost anything. In 1968, a 3M engineer named Spencer Silver invented a light adhesive by accident while working on another project. The adhesive was thought to be useless. After all, who wants glue that sticks, but only just a little? In 1974, Arthur Fye, another 3M employee thought that adhesive would be perfect for holding the bookmark in his hymnal. And the rest is history… Millions of Post-It Notes are sold worldwide where they are used in schools, offices, and houses alike.

This experiment is a method of martial research where not everything discovered will apply. Or perhaps you might find a use for it years later as 3M did with its light adhesive. There may very well be patterns from *macto bicallis* that prove cumbersome, dangerous or that place you in unnecessary risk. Other patterns may work mechanically, but prove counter to your nature. These patterns must be recognized and retooled or discarded.

The Scientific Method

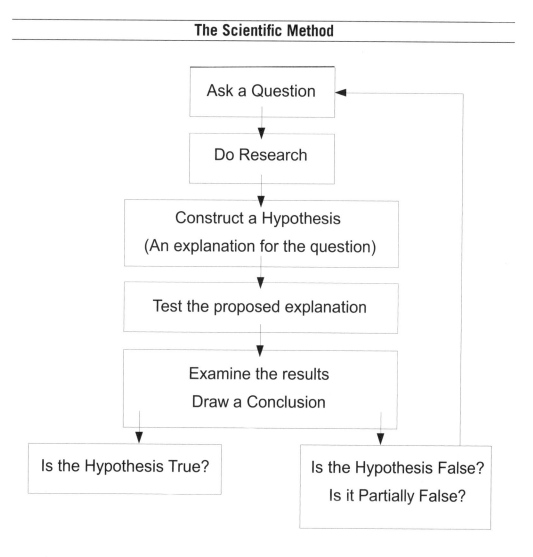

What? I wanna hit people. What's with the geek stuff, Poindexter? Well, a lot actually. The scientific method is important to martial artists, especially those who wish to deeply explore their art. You know, practitioners who can actually use it… for stuff…

The steps of the scientific method are (1) ask a question, (2) do research, (3) construct a hypothesis, (4) test the proposed explanation, (5) examine the results and draw a conclusion, and (6) determine if the hypothesis is true, false, or partially true.

1. Ask a Question

What you're doing is asking a question about something you have observed. You are asking things like how, what, when, who, which, and why. An important aspect of the scientific method is that you have to be able to ask a question that can be measured. It would be nice if the measurement were a number, as it is always the easiest form of information to measure. And it can change over time. For example, ask the question, "How many times can I punch in one second?" However, measurement by numbers is not always possible in the martial arts. If you are fortunate, you will be able to find a situation where you can say something along the lines of, "When I moved my arm this way I was able to hit four times a second as compared to only once."

2. Do Research

This is much simpler than it used to be with the advent of the Internet, Kindle books, videos, email, Twitter, Facebook, and the like, making it possible to communicate instantly with people from across the world. Simply put, the availability and speed of information has never been at the level that it is now. Take advantage of it. Don't start your question from scratch: be smart and don't waste your time.

3. Construct a Hypothesis

That's a fancy phrase for coming up with an educated guess about how something works. If you were to put it in a sentence, it would look like this: "If I do X, then Y will happen." This statement is the center point on which the entire scientific process is based. The challenge is to ensure that your question is asked in a way that can be measured. You also want to make sure that your initial hypothesis is built in such a way as to help you get an answer to your original question. After all, you're trying to become a better fighter here. You want something practical with a measurable result.

4. Test the Proposed Explanation

The construction of your test is important; it needs to be fair and without bias. If you have an agenda with regard to the outcome, then your results are not likely to be as good. To continue with the analogy of punching as many times as you can in one second, let's say you have an instructor, whom you value very profoundly, tell you all a human being is capable of is doing one punch per second. However, you believe that you can do four punches in a second if you hold your elbow a certain way. Your test is constructed in such a way that you have somebody timing you with a stopwatch and you do several repetitions of the first way, confirming that in fact you can get only one punch per second. Then with your elbow held in a certain position you are able to demonstrate repeatedly that you're able to punch four times per second.

5. Examine the Results and Draw a Conclusion

In this instance, you are able to demonstrate that by changing the position of your elbow you are, in fact, able to strike four times per second. Now the issue becomes that somebody I respect and in whom I have invested an enormous amount of time has been proven incorrect. This sort of thing can be emotionally charged and can influence the tester of a hypothesis to make statistical adjustments in response. For example, "Well, those four punches aren't really that hard and wouldn't affect my opponent very much."

Your emotions around the conclusion thus create a thought process that is scientifically incorrect. Let us be specific. You didn't ask how hard you could hit in one second, you asked how many times. Do not allow your agenda or emotions to cloud the information that you have found. The question of how hard can you hit in one second is very different from how many times you can hit in one second. It is important that when engaged in this process, you have clear and distinct parameters for what you are asking, what can be included in your data, information, and results, and what is not to be considered or what is to be excluded.

Further, just because something is excluded does not mean that it is not valid; it simply means that it is not being tested in this format at this time. It's not like you only get one question ever.

6. Is the Hypothesis True?

For the purposes of illustration let us say, "I might believe that I can punch faster and execute more than one punch per second by holding my elbow low and against my side. Is this true?"

7. Is the Hypothesis I am Testing False, or Partially False?

Continuing with our example, the answer is, "My hypothesis is true: I can punch four times a second when I hold my elbow in this position." The other question a tester might raise here would be, "How hard are these punches? If they're just fast but not effective, do they even count?" The answer to that would be that the four punches are technically punches because my fist is closed and I'm striking a pad; further, the "how hard" question was not part of the original hypothesis.

But what if I rephrase the question and create a new hypothesis? "Can I punch more than one time per second hard enough to cause injury to my opponent?" Or "If I punch more than one time per second, (then) I can still cause injury to my opponent." Now that is an entirely different hypothesis that needs to be retested. If you know what your goal is and you know what you want to achieve, then the questions begin to form themselves.

In the case of martial arts, most of us are interested in stopping whatever our opponents are doing to us, as fast as possible. Further, if we select an unarmed art form, such as karate, boxing, or wrestling, more often than not we are using our bodies to make that happen.

So in this example that we have used, one punch per second versus four punches per second is probably not useful for our ultimate goal, which is to make the other person stop what they are doing as fast as possible. There are arguments that could be made that could say, "Well, four punches in a flurry are enough to send somebody into a position of recoil where I can gain advantage." But any scenario based on a flurry of punches starts to become sequentially dependent on anticipated responses and assumed behaviors. That is not always the safest or most efficient route to end a physical altercation in your favor. The potential failure of this tactic is that the success of each movement depends on the success of the previous movement. If any single technique fails, the whole sequence won't work.

As you go through *macto bicallis*, it is essential that you apply the scientific method. Apply the method stringently and with emphasis toward simplicity. It might sound like a lot of work, but if you go through the process you will undoubtedly become a better fighter, be it in the ring or on the street. The starting point is discovering your fighting nature. From there you can build a repertoire that is natural, instinctive, and successful.

Finding the Fighter's Nature

There are three basic fighting natures: striking, grappling, and running (which also include the subsets "runner to" and "runner from" the danger). No one person is totally one singular nature. Every person has a dominant and a secondary fighting nature. It is possible that there is also a tertiary nature; however, we believe that focusing on the dominant and secondary nature is sufficient to help you train to take advantage of your strengths and minimize your weaknesses.

It is also important to know that the context of an incident can change a person's dominant fighting nature, or it can remain the same. An example of this might be the "cornered rat." The cornered rat concept says that a rat trapped, with no other options, will fight to the death no matter the size of the aggressor. Sun Tzu addresses this in *The Art of War* and recommends giving an opponent an avenue to escape. Battling an opponent who has nothing to lose is an expensive proposition, even if you prevail. A person with a primary nature of runner, once trapped, may switch to a striker personality under the cornered rat scenario.

> *"Soldiers when in desperate straits lose the sense of fear. If there is no place of refuge, they will stand firm. If they are in hostile country, they will show a stubborn front. If there is no help for it, they will fight hard."*
>
> —Sun Tzu, The Art of War (Section 24)

It is also possible that their primary nature of runner is so dominant that they cannot see other options, even when trapped with no place to run. In this instance, unable to run, their brain freezes and submits to the threat.

Finding Your Fighting Nature: A Test

These tests take some effort to make them successful. Front loading or tipping off the test subject must be avoided to the extent possible as it risks creating a false result. It is also important to note that these are field tests; they are not perfect. They are, however, designed to produce quick, reasonable results that you can act on.

You will need the following:

1. Three people: the test subject, the controller, and the target.
2. A whistle or some means of making a loud shocking sound to begin the test.

The test is performed this way. The test subject begins doing jumping jacks. The controller will blow the whistle unexpectedly at some random time. At that moment, the test subject must instantly turn and attack his training partner, the target. This will be done five times.

See the grid.

Macto Bicallis Fighting Tendency Grid

	1	2	3	4	5	Total
Grappler						
Run to						
Striker						
Run from						

The target stands behind the subject knowing that he or she is going to be attacked. We highly recommend the test be done with the target wearing padding and a helmet, something like a Redman, Bulletman, Gort (shown below), or High Gear suit for safety.

The test subject, however, does not wear any form of padding. This is to ensure as natural a response as possible since in a real-world experience these pads will not be present. Now, clearly, the introduction of padding on the target changes some aspects of the testing, but to operate without these safety measures places the target at unnecessary risk without doing anything to help find the test subject's fighting nature.

You will do the test five times. It is important to randomize, the easiest method of which is to create a lottery. Simply write 1, 2, 3, 4, and 5 on slips of paper. These five numbers represent the five positions on the floor from which the target will begin each attack.

Have the target draw one number and then assume the position on the floor that the number indicates. It is important that the test subject has his or her back turned and be in position to begin the test at this point so as not to see the target's position. Furthermore, the subject has begun his jumping jacks to help obfuscate the positioning of the target.

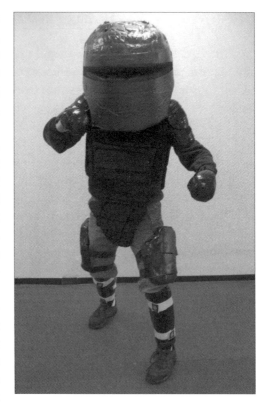

Once everyone is in position, the controller stands back and blows the whistle loudly and with intent to disturb the test subject. It is best to time the whistle while the subject is in the air. At that signal, the subject must turn and attack the target instantly, no hesitation should be allowed.

As the controller, you need to watch what the subject chooses to use to attack his target. As an example, if he chooses to grab, it means he is a grappler. If he chooses to push the target to the ground, then you would mark the subject as a striker. For the purposes of this test, pushes and shoves should be categorized as strikes. The focus for the controller needs to be on the initial contact only, not any follow-on techniques. This is because the first movement is the one least likely to be influenced by higher brain functions, hence the best indicator of the fighter's nature.

After each test run, record what the subject did. At the end of the five trials, add up the results. The majority tells you the fighter's tendency. For example, 3 grapples and 2 strikes would be identified as a grappler with striking undertones. Five strikes equal a heavy preference to striking. You may even find that you have 3 strikes and 2 runs or something similar.

Notes on Running to/from

Again, understand that it is rare that any person has only one fighting nature. However, his training can lead to such a behavior. As an example, a high school wrestler is going to default to his training and throw everybody to the ground; a boxer will try to strike with his hands. A person's training will clearly influence his choices, even to the point of taking a long and inefficient route to make the moment conform to his preferred methods of fighting. Sometimes the preferred tool is not the right tool for the job, and a quick grab from the metaphorical tool box will bring better results.

Choosing a style that fits well with your fighting nature is important because your training will augment your natural preferences, yet it is also important to look at the holes in your training and not get overly locked in on "predefined" solutions. For example, while running is often better than fighting, especially when your goal is escape, few practitioners actively train to do that. The same goes for verbal de-escalation and situational awareness. Most everyone knows that those skills are important, but few practice them as diligently as they do striking or grappling.

One final example: A target that untrained combatants naturally take to is hair. Pulling an adversary's hair causes pain, helps you gain control the other guy's body, and often places you in a position of tactical advantage when higher levels of force are necessary. But, most "trained" martial artists never even think about trying it in a fight. That's because hair pulling is outlawed in martial sports and is rarely considered a viable target in martial arts. What gets trained gets done.

Running carries with it a certain stigma that is not based in reality. We find knights screaming, "Run away! Run away!" in the classic movie, *Monty Python and the Holy Grail*. Screaming, running knights is funny because it appears overtly cowardly yet the knights of history were not cowards. Running is considered in some ways a less than favorable way to deal with a situation. But the fact is that running keeps people alive, especially running from a superior threat. Simply put, running is a serious and valid form of self-defense. The only fight you are guaranteed to win is the one you never engage in. If you're not there, the other guy can't hit you.

Put this in your head: running is a good idea. Not always, but often enough. File it away and plan on using that tactic when appropriate (e.g., the other guy has a knife or gun, or there are more threats than there are of you, to name a few instances where retreat is prudent).

The Techniques and Degrees of Force

While strikes can be used in a drunkle situation, unless you are very skilled and experienced, it is generally a good idea to use them only in sport or combat. After all, if you damage your spouse's favorite uncle after he's had few too many at the family picnic, you'll be sleeping on the couch for a long time. Or worse…

Striking in sports typically involves protective hand gear. Gloves soften the impact and help assure that, win or lose; participants can fight again another day. Without this equipment, you can cause more or less damage by altering the target, angle, or force with which you strike. Any blow to the head or neck can be severely disabling, potentially leading to long-term injury or death. That's a felony if you do it under the wrong circumstances. Be cautious about where and how you hit on the street.

Commonly, four areas affect damage:

1. Angle—There are many vital areas on the human body, places that are easier to break, such as the eyes, neck, or solar plexus, when compared to the thigh, back, or buttocks. If you have been practicing martial arts for a while you should already know where these weak areas are. What you may not realize is that the angle of attack contributes hugely to the damage. For example, a horizontal eye-rake versus a straight-in jab/displacement; the former is oftentimes easier to perform yet the latter can cause significantly more injury.

2. Intensity—This is a combination of speed, strength, and body alignment. For example, if you relax your body when you throw a punch, even hold your fist loosely, and then tense everything at the moment of impact, you will hit a lot harder than if you keep your muscles tight the entire way. This is because the first method moves much faster than the second. But, if you don't align your body properly at the moment of impact, much of the force will bleed off, lessening the blow. If the speed of your blow remains constant, it becomes a push; whereas, if it accelerates through the moment of impact, it is a strike.

3. Weapon—In unarmed conflict, the weapon is typically your head, teeth, shoulders, elbows, fists, hips, knees, or legs, but even amongst those choices you have sub-options. For example, do you slap with an open hand or hit with a closed fist? You can also use areas like your chest to damage an adversary's limb by bridging the joint across it. Of course, you can bring foreign objects into play: "found" things like rocks, sticks, bottles, pool cues, or "designed" things like batons, knives, or guns,

to increase the odds of delivering debilitating damage. Don't forget that you don't always have to use the object to strike the other guy; you can also use your adversary to strike the object. Shoving an adversary in front of a moving vehicle, down a stairwell, or into wall can mess him up pretty bad.

4. Striking area—These attacks refer not only to the part of the body you strike, but also to how you impact it. For example, slapping the solar plexus with an open hand has far less impact than a closed fist, even with the same intensity of blow. This is because the palm spreads the impact over a wider surface area. Similarly, a single knuckle strike does even more than the fist when attacking that same spot because it focuses the energy into a very small area (much like driving a nail into a board). You can use contouring to hit any vital area with the most (or least) effective weapon in order to control damage.

Grappling naturally lends itself fairly well to the various levels of force. But it can be hazardous. Throwing a guy who doesn't know how to fall properly can lead to unintended consequences such as a broken neck. So can spending time on the ground. Before you go down, be certain that the other guy does not have friends nearby who will put the boots to you. And don't hang out there. Do what you need to do and get back up quickly.

Real life isn't a tournament; there are no referees and few rules. Sure, society has codified a ginormous set of laws governing violence, but for all practical purposes, in any given fight (other than the laws of physics) those rules are in somebody's head. During that physical confrontation, it's damnably tough to know if the other guy is playing by the same rules you are. You may never know until it's too late. You can't control him, but you can control you. You decide what you're going to attempt to do, how you're going to do it, and what type of damage you are striving for.

Keep in mind that while pain hurts, damage lasts. A pressure point, armbar, or Taser® can convince someone to change their behavior, yet there is rarely any lasting injury resulting from proper application of these techniques (assuming you can call a Taser a technique). Assuming they work. More often than not, pain alone is insufficient to stop a determined attacker. Damage, on the other hand, includes such things as broken bones, internal injuries, loss of consciousness, or similar trauma that results in extended hospitalization (all of which tend to be found in definitions of felony assault). The situation you find yourself in and the person(s) you face will dictate the appropriate response.

Over the next several pages, we will demonstrate several common techniques, showing how they work in competition, drunkle, and combative encounters. This is by no means a holistic appraisal of the numerous techniques out there, but there are enough examples for you to understand the principles and make prudent decisions about applying whatever it is that you study in the ring or using it on the street.

Don't try to simply memorize the differences in application between techniques designed to win a tournament, wrangle a drunk, or destroy an enemy. Instead, strive to understand the reason for these variations so that you can incorporate them into your martial art, train hard, and make them your own.

Arms and Hands

The following techniques tend to come most naturally to the striker. In general, it is best to hit hard things (e.g., chin) with soft things (e.g., palm heel) and vice versa. Hitting hard to hard (e.g., knuckle to chin) hurts and can cause damage to the striker, never a good thing in a fight. This is particularly important to remember if you practice an art where gloves are commonplace (e.g., boxing, MMA) and you find yourself having to perform these applications on the street. If you don't align your knuckles, wrist, and arm properly, you are liable to break something. It's tough to fight when it's excruciatingly painful to use your hands, so practice with a heavy bag, *makiwara*, or other solid surface (under proper supervision) without gloves until you can do it naturally.

When performed by a skilled practitioner, some of the techniques below can prove fatal or severely disabling. Use prudence when using them on another human being. For strikes, the main differences between sport, drunkle, and combat applications are which targets you choose, what weapon you apply (e.g., open hand vs. closed fist), the angle of attack, and how intensely (and often) you strike. Nevertheless, most strikes tend to fit sport and combat applications better than drunkle scenarios.

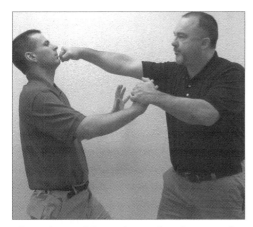 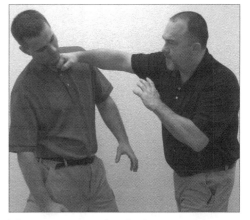

The jab is delivered to the face in this instance, and, in particular, the chin. By twisting the torso slightly, the jab is extended to get more reach, allowing contact with the adversary and hopefully keeping your body out of striking range. The target is often the face, jaw, or eye socket.

The cross is considered a heavy punch, usually used in combination as a follow-up to a jab. It is called a cross because it crosses the centerline of the person throwing the punch. The heaviness of the punch comes from the twisting of the body and the shifting of the bodyweight forward. The target is usually the side of the head.

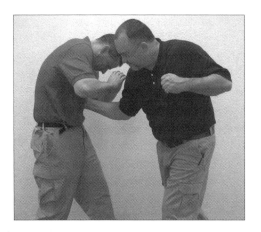

The inside uppercut is a close range technique that uses the upward momentum of the fist and snapping of the punching shoulder forward to explode the striking fist upward into the adversary. Common targets can be the chin or the solar plexus.

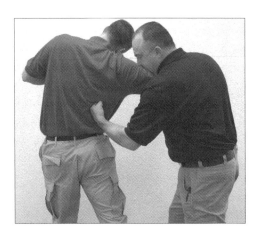

The outside uppercut delivered to the outside line of the adversary contains all the aspects of the inside uppercut—the upward momentum of the fist and the snapping and dropping of the striking shoulder. The favored target is the floating ribs, and, on the right side of the attacker, the liver.

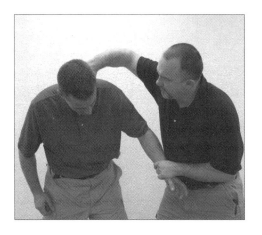

The roundhouse punch is a close range technique designed to go around the forward defenses of the opponent. In this instance, we are using a left grab to prevent the adversary from blocking and/or moving out of the way of the strike. The targets for this strike are usually the side of the head or jaw. In this instance, the target is the back side of the neck.

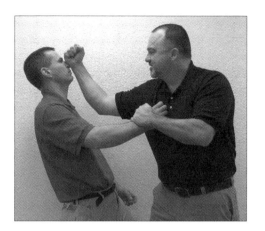

The hammerfist is delivered in a downward arch, as if swinging a hammer at a nail. The name is also derived from the fist being used in the same way as a hammer is used; the fist mimics a hammer. The targets for this technique are many; in this instance, it is the nose/face of the adversary. The side of the hand is soft, facilitating strikes to hard areas of the opponent with less chance of injury while still delivering significant force.

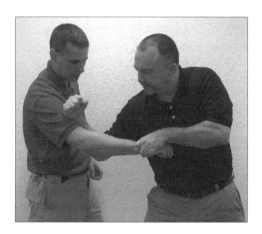

The forearm smash to the biceps is done by drawing the striking forearm across your own body, striking the adversary's far arm; in other words, your right forearm to the other guy's right biceps. Your fist twists at impact, smashing the larger of the two forearm bones, the ulna, into the adversary's biceps. This blow is designed to incapacitate the arm via muscle damage and is an immediate precursor to another technique of your choice.

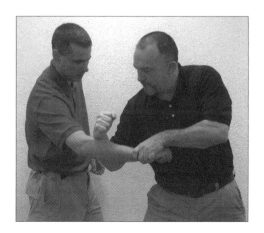

The forearm smash to the adversary's forearm is done in the same manner as the forearm smash to the biceps. This strike often pulls the opponent forward, while inflicting pain. Once again, this is not a finishing technique and is used to gain advantage and inflict pain.

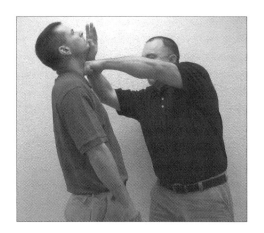

The fist to the adversary's throat strike is a straight punch to the throat. In this instance, the right hand is used to clear the chin and deliver the strike directly to the trachea. This technique can cause very severe injuries; use it only when the tactical situation requires it.

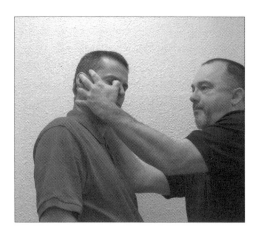

The bear claw attack to the throat is done in the same manner as the straight punch; however, this time the fist is configured for a bear claw strike using the middle joints of the fingers. This strike is a smaller profile fist, often a more viable option than a traditional fore fist as it contours to the target area more effectively. Once again, this attack is very dangerous, so use it wisely.

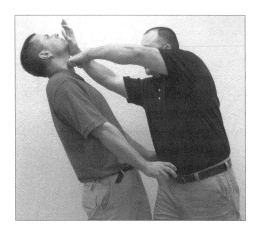

When inserting the thumb into the eye, use the side of the nose as a brace and push the thumb into the eye socket. This is not a tear or gouge, but a displacement. The thumb serves a wedge to damage the eye. Street fighters and thugs often have long, sharpened thumbnails to facilitate this application. Eye strikes are tremendously serious. While hugely disabling when performed correctly, they will cause massive retaliation if they fail. Be prudent with this.

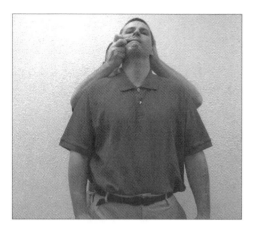

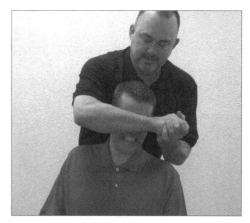

The fishhook can be done using one or more fingers. The goal is to pull the cheek of the adversary controlling the head and turning it by pulling the inside of the cheek. It doesn't necessarily cause damage in and of itself, but if the adversary feels pain, it does facilitate other follow-on applications that will. And there's a certain degree of mechanical leverage. When you are able to control the other guy's head, the rest of his body is much easier to manage.

In the cross face strike done from behind, in a standing or ground position, the ulna of the arm is placed across the bridge of the nose. You use your body to brace the back of the adversary's head to reduce movement and potential escape. Both arms are used to draw the right arm's ulna into the adversary's face. Rotating the arm up and down by twisting the right wrist will create more pain. Be aware that techniques performed from behind an adversary require a lot of justification should you find yourself having to explain what you did in court. A key question the prosecutor will ask is "If you were able to get behind him, why couldn't you simply run away?"

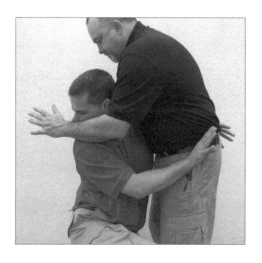

In wrestling competition, the cross face technique is taught from the back. The adversary is face down on the ground and you are lying on his back, head-to-head, feet-to-feet. The principles are the same in this instance except it is done to the front. Start with your left hand close to your stomach and push the nose of your opponent to the left. Grind the radius bone of your arm across the adversary's face turning their head with intent to clasp your hand behind their head.

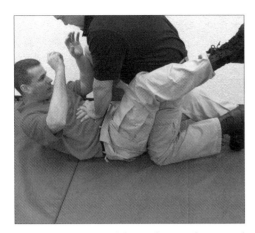

The gut pump is delivered in a downward angle and toward the shoulder blades from the front side of the body by compressing the hands on the xiphoid process and driving in a sharp, deep, and explosive thrust.

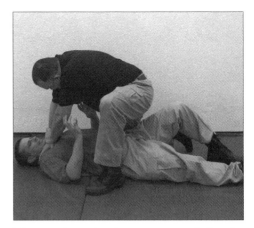

This attack to the throat is not a choke; the intent is to crush the larynx. The right hand is placed on the front of the throat, similar to a karate knife hand; the left hand grabs the right hand to aid in support and focuses your bodyweight into the adversary's throat. This is done with a sharp thrust and then pressure is applied. It's potentially deadly. Even if the initial damage doesn't prove fatal, swelling can cut off oxygen if medical treatment is not quickly forthcoming. Don't use this one lightly.

Head

While you don't naturally want to get hit in the head during a fight, sometimes the head makes a useful tool to smash the other guy with. Anyone who has played soccer knows how powerfully you can strike with your forehead, yet pretty much anything around the "hat band" line works. Just don't lead with your face. Such techniques are pretty ubiquitous in Europe and South America, but for some reason are not nearly as popular in the United States, hence can sometimes catch an adversary by surprise.

The trick to making head butts work without hurting yourself is not only to be careful about what part of the head you strike with, but also to assure that you use your body rather than your neck to do it. We like to think of it as bowing aggressively. Augmenting the strike with a grab can make it even more effective (e.g., the infamous "Glasgow kiss") because the adversary cannot easily get out of the way. When grabbed from behind, a reverse head butt can sometimes be effective as well.

As with other strikes, the targets you choose, angle of attack, and intensity will determine application. Head butts are illegal in many, but not all martial sports. A blow to the adversary's chest can set up a takedown or throw for a drunkle encounter; whereas a similar strike to his face might cause combat-worthy damage. Nevertheless, this is something you're more likely to try in combat than in either a sporting or drunkle scenario.

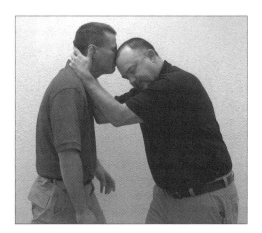

The head butt can be a powerful strike. In this example, you use your hands to secure the neck of the adversary. This stance is not essential for success; however, the combination of pulling and driving your head into the face increases the striking force. Notice you turn your face slightly away using the side of your frontal bone to make contact with the adversary.

Legs and Feet

While most strikers can naturally throw punches, hitting with the legs, feet, and knees takes a bit of training. Timing and balance are also important here, as whenever you lift your leg to strike you simultaneously lose your balance, albeit temporarily if you do it right. If you are wearing boots, the position of the foot is less important than if you perform the techniques barefoot or while wearing soft shoes, in which case it's important to avoid (painfully) jamming your toes into the adversary. If your foot becomes damaged or the opponent captures your leg when you attempt a kick, you may lose the opportunity to run away, even when you really, really need to.

If you stomp someone in a street fight, plan on having to justify your actions in court. Such things may be necessary and legitimate, but they have a tendency to look like excessive force (especially when caught on camera and played before a jury).

As with any strike, differences between sport, drunkle, and combat applications are which targets you choose, the angle of attack, and how intensely (and often) you strike. In some sports, padded footwear is required. For street applications, what you are wearing can make a difference between drunkle and combat. For example, a padded high-top (e.g., basketball shoe) is likely to cause a lot less damage than a steel-toed boot regardless of where you strike. Nevertheless, this stuff tends to fit sport and combat applications better than drunkle scenarios.

For skilled practitioners, some of the techniques below can prove lethal or permanently disabling, so this is another of those "don't do this at home" kind of things… unless your life is on the line and you are prepared to justify it before a judge and jury.

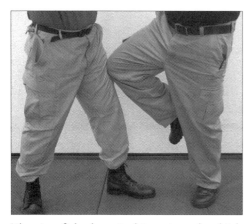

The tip of the knee is driven into the thigh muscles of the adversary. The goal of this strike is bruising and muscle damage, to make your adversary's use of his leg painful. It's a good technique to facilitate your ability to disengage and run away.

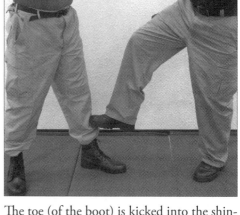

The toe (of the boot) is kicked into the shinbone (tibia) of the adversary in an explosive, short, and painful strike. This kick is virtually impossible to block. It can be evaded, of course, but only if seen. Used in combination with a punch to the face it can be easy to obfuscate. The kick's goal is to inflict pain and elicit a retreating step from the adversary.

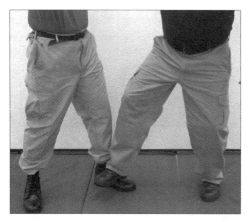

Use the heel of your foot to stomp downward on the arch of the foot with intent to displace the bones (cuneiform and metatarsals) from their normal position rendering the foot damaged and difficult to use without pain. Again, this is a great way to slow down an adversary so that you can get away.

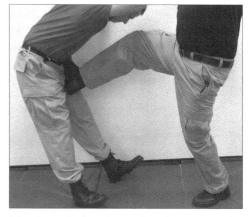

The thrust kick is directed to the groin or the stomach, as in the *pankration gastrizein*, with intent to do as much damage as possible and blow the opponent backward away from the person who executed the kick. The non-kicking or "base" foot should be planted firmly on the ground, while the kicking foot snaps forward from the knee and into the adversary, the hips and base foot delivering the push.

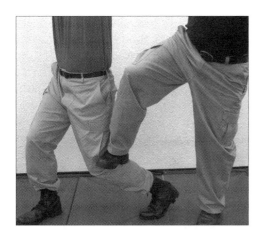

The intent of this knee kick technique is to tear the tendons of the knee while causing it to collapse and become useless for mobility. Done right, it takes surgery and rehabilitation before the victim can use the joint properly again. The usual attack to the knee is done as shown, from outside to inside, although there are other options as well. Kicks to the front of the knee don't typically cause as much damage as those that come in from the side or back.

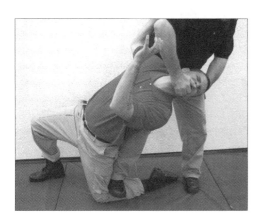

Stomping on the back of the knee drives the adversary's kneecap (patella) into the ground, the harder the ground the greater the potential for damage. Standing on the knee, pins it to the ground and allows for other follow-up attacks. This view of the knee stomp demonstrates high/low manipulation of the adversary's body. This is harder to thwart than a kick alone. Any combination that disrupts an adversary's structure makes it easier to cause damage with a follow-on strike.

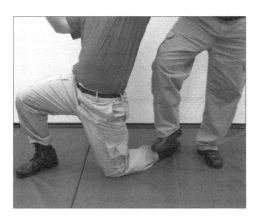

The ankle stomp is a very powerful technique from a strategic and tactical standpoint, one that can facilitate escape. The ankle is comprised of several small bones that allow for a high level of mobility. The ends of the fibula, tibia from the upper leg, meeting the talus, calcaneus, and cuboid, and to some extent, the navicular and the cuneiforms, can be knocked out of position tearing the ligaments that hold the bones in place (the anterior and posterior tibiotalar, as well as the tibionavicular and the tibioncalcaneal ligaments). This is a very powerful technique from a strategic and tactical stand point, one that can facilitate escape.

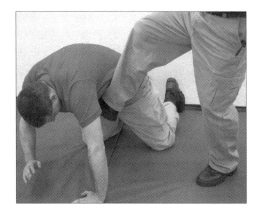

The target of the rib kick is the floating ribs; these ribs are only attached to the spine and do not attach to the sternum. You can use the tip of a boot or the top of the foot. One way to think about this is the difference between kickers in the National Football League. Placekickers tend to use the tip of their shoe while punters use the top of their foot. For our purposes, either is acceptable. Concentrate on moving swiftly and pulling the leg back immediately after contact so that you can regain your balance and mobility while evading capture of your striking leg.

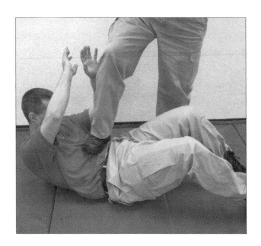

The abdomen stomp is not a sophisticated technique. Simply put, stomp downward onto your adversary's abdomen. The intent is to cause damage to the internal organs. But, as mentioned previously, stomping on a downed opponent doesn't tend to play well in court. Make sure you can articulate why this was necessary.

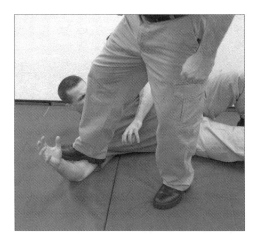

Without a fulcrum, it is difficult to break a bone in the adversary's arm when it is flat on the ground. The intent of arm stomp is to crush soft tissue, veins, arteries, and muscle. Downward stomp, "helpless" victim, be justified and all that…

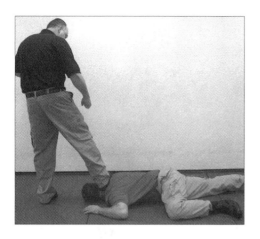

Delivered to the back of the neck, the stomp is designed to crush the cervical vertebra and has the potential to sever the spinal column. This stomp can be deadly, particularly if the victim is lying across a curb or similar surface. Use it only where warranted.

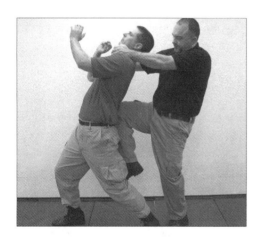

Pulling the shoulders backward, the knee is driven into the lower back with intent to create pain and to break the adversary's balance for a follow-up technique.

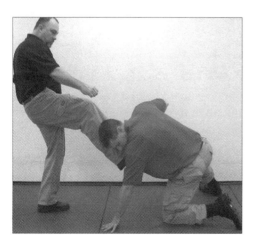

When the adversary is on the ground, especially with all fours on the ground, the same kick that is used in the rib kick is used on the face of the other guy. Kicking to the face/head of a standing adversary is bound to fail unless you achieve total surprise or are far faster or more skilled than the other guy. When he's on the ground, not so much. But it can cause very serious damage and must be done only when prudent.

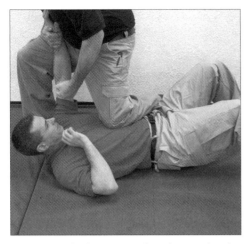

Dropping the knee onto the adversary's solar plexus, or sternum with full force and bodyweight, the pin is designed to allow for follow-up techniques.

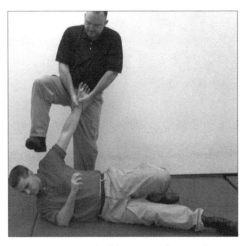

Having a secure hold on an adversary's arm, use your back to pull upward in a swift and sharp motion.

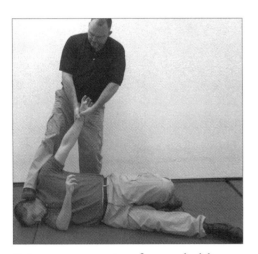

Raise your stomping foot and deliver a stomp to the head while pulling upward on the other guy's arm.

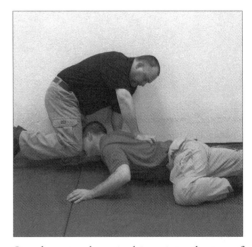

Simply put, a knee is driven into the top of the adversary's head or in this case the face if the other guy looks up. Take note of the pinning action of the hands on the back of the adversary to restrict escape routes. Note that should the adversary cover his head with his hands, you can still strike through the hands or arms. Again, this can cause very serious damage, so use it wisely.

Small Joint Manipulations

Small joint (e.g., fingers, toes) manipulations are illegal in virtually all sporting events because of the potential for injury. But you will rarely tangle with a barefoot adversary, and even if you do, hands are easier to get at than feet, so we'll focus on fingers. In a real fight, this is an area that warrants attention, both to control an adversary as well as to make him let go of you or a weapon. For example, law enforcement officers and security personnel routinely use finger locks to augment come-along holds, restraints, and hand-cuffing techniques. The challenge is that during a fast and furious fight, especially in an adrenalized state, these little buggers can be damnably tough to latch onto. Nevertheless, there are a plethora of techniques designed to exploit the fingers (and thumb) as weak points. By adjusting the intensity, you can use the following techniques for either drunkle or combat applications.

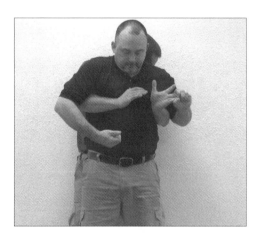

Peel the finger(s) backward against the joint. By rotating the wrist, you can increase the angle of the attack, increase pain, and possibly dislocate the fingers more swiftly.

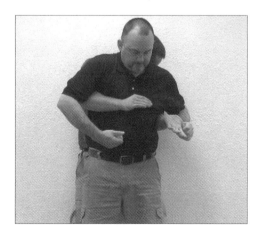

The strongest member of the hand, the thumb, is most difficult to dislocate. However, it can serve as a lever to manipulate the hand and the arm. This mechanical leverage can be used to imbalance or disrupt the adversary and set up follow-on techniques that cause damage.

Grappling Techniques in Sport, Drunkle, and Combat

As mentioned previously, grappling techniques more naturally offer variations appropriate for sporting, drunkle, and combative applications than strikes do. However, in drunkle or combat situations, you will often need a disruption, such as a strike, to set up your technique for success, which is why we covered them first. After all, it's extremely hard to walk up to an actively resisting adversary and slap a lock, hold, or throw on him. The selection that follows will take you through various examples of techniques, demonstrating modifications that allow them to work at all three levels of force.

One additional thing to note is the fighting surface. In a tournament, you'll be tossing the other guy onto a padded structure, be it a traditional *tatami* mat, "squared circle," or octagon ring. On the street, not so much—at minimum the landing area won't be padded. Potentially, it will be downright dangerous (e.g., landing on broken glass, discarded needles, sharp rocks, or other debris). The same thing goes for a barroom floor or even your own living room (unless you have an awfully thick carpet and no furniture). What the adversary lands on may do as much if not more damage than the technique you used to put him there. Be mindful of this.

Particularly in the drunkle scenario, it may be prudent to control the other guy's fall by holding onto him and guiding him, if not gently at least not jarringly, to the ground. This isn't just because of what he may be falling onto, but also due to how he may fall. Accidently breaking the neck or dislocating the shoulder of someone who doesn't know how to land correctly would not be a good thing. On purpose, sure, if that's your goal (e.g., combat), but not by mistake. But there's danger in doing the nice guy thing too. The tactical circumstances will help you decide. In general, if the other guy is drunk and the skill differential is high, this kinder, gentler approach will work out well.

Osoto Gari

Osoto gari is translated as "major outer reaping throw." It has, with little doubt, been around since the first caveman tripped his buddy throwing him to the ground. It is classified by the judo canon, devised by judo's founder Jigoro Kano, as one of the original 40 throws. *Osoto gari* has a long tradition of success; nearly every *judoka* has used it in competition, so it is one of the sport's fundamentals.

The reason that it works so well is that it's simple. You break your opponent's posture, hook his leg, and hurl him backward onto the ground with force. Pretty sweet, huh? But, it's a double-edged sword. Your stance must be strong and your adversary's weak, or it will be easy for him to counter, using precisely that same throw. In order to succeed, you will need to disrupt his posture before executing the technique.

For a bit of finesse, turn your hips rather than going straight back like a "tippy bird" as you cut his leg and you will increase your chances of success.

Osoto Gari—Competition

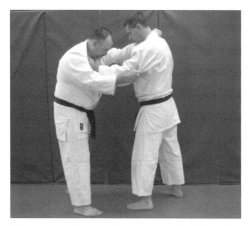

Using a modern judo grip, one hand on the collar and the other on the elbow, and then engage your opponent.

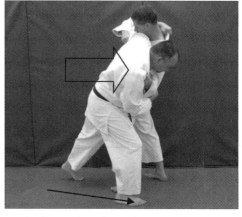

Dash forward and to the outside of your opponent, planting your right foot while simultaneously breaking his balance. This obviously can be done to either side; we're only showing one example.

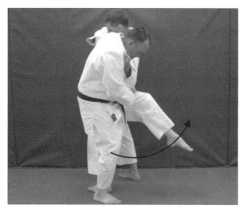

Lift your left leg high and behind your opponent's left leg in preparation to sweep, or cut the opponent's leg out from underneath him.

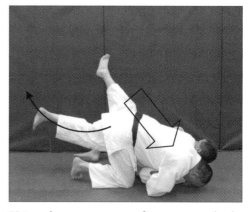

Using the momentum of your upper body, drive the opponent to the ground as you cut his left leg from underneath him.

Osoto Gari—Drunkle

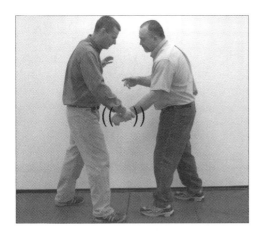

Securing your adversary's left arm, in this instance with a grab, prepare to drive inward toward the opponent.

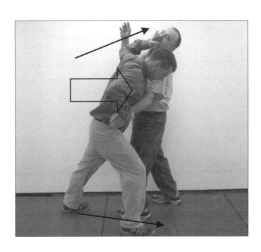

Step aggressively forward with the right foot; drive your left palm upward under the adversary's jaw, pushing his head backward. Controlling the head in this fashion makes the rest of his body follow. This isn't legal in competition, but softening up the other guy with a blow makes virtually any throw easier to pull off.

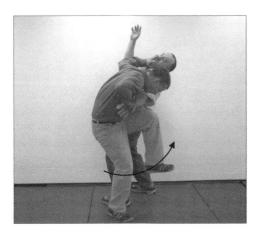

Continue to drive forward lifting the left leg with intent to cut the adversary's left leg out from under him.

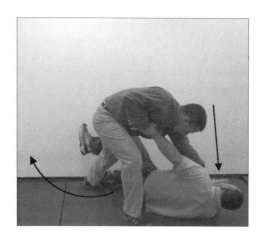

Drive your adversary to the ground with the combination of the sweeping of his left leg and the palm of the left hand pushing his head backward. Avoid going to the ground with the other guy; you can do damage by falling on him and, unless you need to follow up with a pin, it's tactically superior to be standing when he's not.

Osoto Gari—Combat

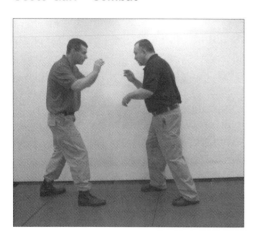

You and your attacker are face-to-face and you are seeking an opportunity to grab or deflect the attackers left hand, arm, or in this instance, his wrist.

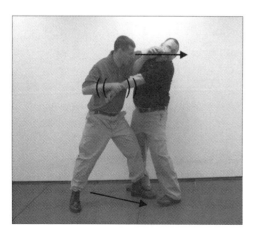

Reach out with your right hand and grab the attacker's left wrist. Step in with your left foot and drive your left arm into his face. When we say left arm, we need everything from little finger to the elbow, using the hand and lower arm as a battering ram. At this point, the attacker will most likely attempt to block your right forearm. It makes little difference. The key to the forearm motion is to ensure that the attacker has been forced back on his heels, compromising his balance.

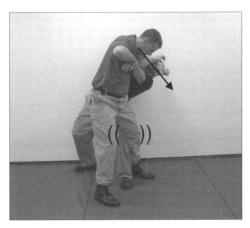

As with the other versions of *osoto gari*, you step across with your left leg. However, in this modification you drive your leg downward into the back or into the side of the attacker's left knee.

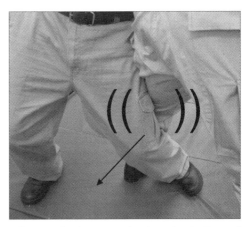

Observe the knees are back to back. Extend the back of your knee into your attacker's leg bending his knee. Your heel needs to be on the same line as your attacker's heel or deeper.

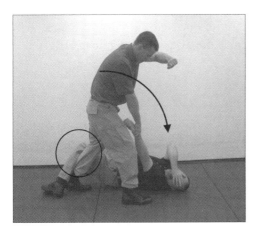

Having used a combination of the collapsed support of the leg and the forearm to the face to drive the attacker to the ground, make every attempt to remain standing.

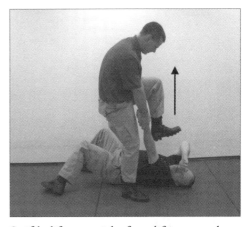

Swiftly lift your right foot, lifting your knee high. You are now using both hands to hold the attacker's left arm.

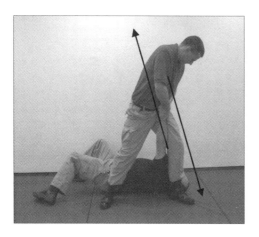

Simultaneously pull upward with both hands on the attacker's left arm while stomping down into the face with the left foot. While this is effective, it's not going to look good to a jury. Be certain that you can justify this in court before attempting this technique.

Ko Uchi Gari

Ko uchi gari is a small, inner reaping throw, another staple of judo. There is a tendency to go to the ground with your opponent, so care must be taken to assure that you land in an advantageous position for any follow-on grappling necessary afterward. And keeping with the ongoing theme and recommendation, all grappling must be kept to a minimum with the ultimate goal of regaining your feet as soon as possible. Unless, of course, you are in a sports competition or your goal is to control the other guy until help arrives and it is safe to do so.

Ko Uchi Gari—Competition

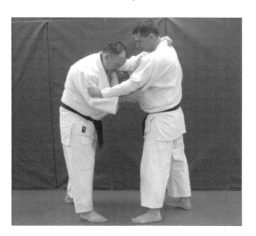

Using a traditional judo grip, left hand high on the collar and right hand on the elbow, tie up with your opponent.

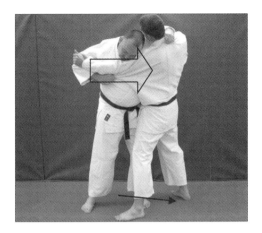

Pinning the opponent's left arm with your right arm, step in with your left foot to make contact from your head down to your waist. The intent of this contact is to drive the opponent backward, disrupting his balance.

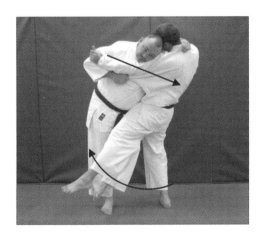

Driving your opponent backward to remove his bodyweight from his left foot, use your left foot to clip the back heel of your opponent's left foot, sweeping your leg across your centerline and in the direction of his toes. It is important that you try not to move your opponent straight back, but rather work for roughly 45 degrees to your right, essentially where his foot used to be.

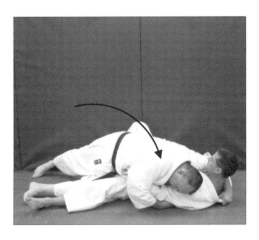

Land on your opponent staying tight and leaving no space between your two bodies, which holds your dominant position. This position allows you to move directly into groundwork should you not score an *ippon* ending the match.

Ko Uchi Gari—Drunkle

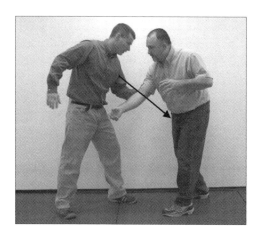

As the adversary reaches with his right hand, meet his arm at the elbow with your hand in a sweeping motion across his body.

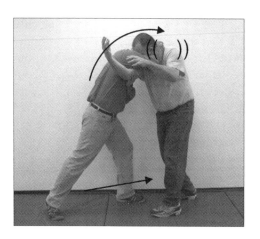

Shift in with your left foot to close distance and with your right arm wrap up the adversary's head, reaching deep behind and to the back of the other guy's back with intent to control his head as tightly as possible.

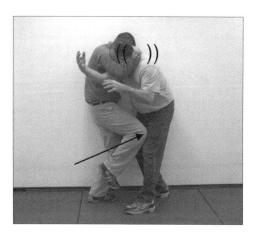

Strike with your knee at the left side of the adversary while pulling his head in tightly. Although the groin is a possible target, the thigh is used to make the adversary step back.

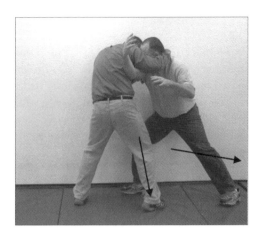

As the adversary steps back with his left leg, place your right foot down, seeking the centerline and center space between your two bodies.

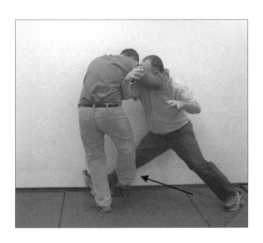

With your right foot powerfully sweep the back of the adversary's right forward leg, lifting his heel and sweeping forward.

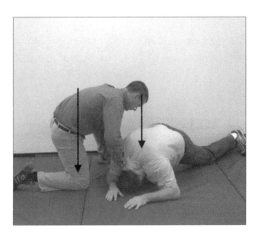

Stepping back with your right foot, drop to your right knee. With your left hand in the armpit of the adversary pulling forward, keep your right hand on the back of the other guy's head bringing him forward at a 45-degree angle. Slam him face down into the ground leaving you in the dominant position. Be cautious about what you drop the other guy onto in a drunkle situation so that you do not cause unintended damage. It is very challenging for the other guy to break his fall properly when thrown this way.

Ko Uchi Gari—Combat

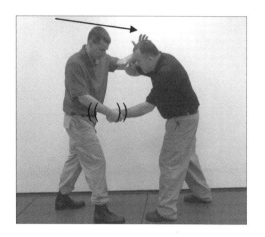

As you face off with the attacker, use your right hand to grab the attacker's left arm (or in this instance wrist). Simultaneously strike the right side of the attacker's head with your open palm. This may seem less effective than a closed-fist punch, but done properly it can cause sufficient damage and disorientation without the inherent risk of hurting yourself by striking with a closed fist. And it looks better for witnesses too.

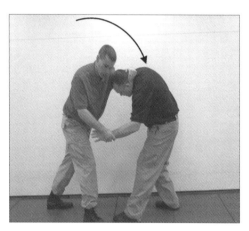

Wrapped behind the attacker's neck with your left hand bringing as much weight as you can, bend him over and force his weight onto his left foot, immobilizing it for a split second.

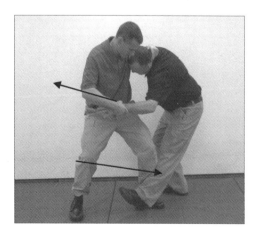

Drive your left shin into the other guy's knee with intent to collapse it. Simultaneously pull his right hand to your hip, increasing the weight on his left leg.

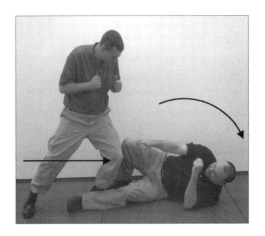

Having pulled down on the neck and collapsed his knee, use your left arm to pull the attacker's head down and push forward at the same time, driving him to the ground. Once he begins to fall, release the other guy and let him crash to the ground on his own accord. It is far better to remain on your feet if you can than it is to follow him onto the ground. Letting go will actually increase the damage he takes when he falls.

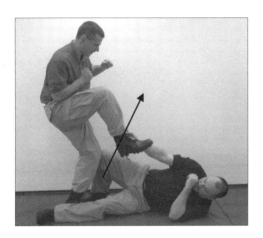

Step up the left foot, lifting your knee high with intent to stomp on any available target. In this instance, the attacker's face is available.

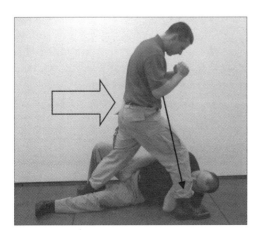

Drive forward placing as much weight as possible downward and into your stomp. This is a simultaneous forward and downward stomping motion. And, of course, you need to be able to justify it in court.

Osoto Gake

Osoto gake can be thought of as a long-range version of *osoto gari*. It translates as "major outer hooking throw." The basic movements and mechanics between these two throws are similar, breaking the other guy's balance and putting him on his back. The difference is the distance between the two people. *Osoto gari* is closer while *osoto gake* works from farther away. It can be executed on an opponent whose legs are too far away for an *osoto gari* attack, or after a failed *osoto gari* as a recovery/follow-on technique, or where the other guy has stepped backward to escape your initial attack. Having both a short- and a long-game adds flexibility for dealing with a rapidly moving threat.

Osoto Gake—Competition

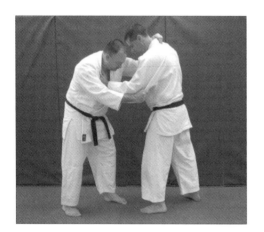

From a traditional judo grip, left hand high on the collar and right hand on the opponent's elbow, pull your opponent forward and slightly downward.

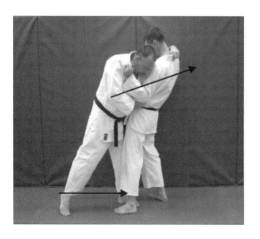

As you feel your opponent fight the pull forward, dash inward with a left foot shuffle. This should accelerate the movement that the other guy began of his own accord and drive your opponent backward.

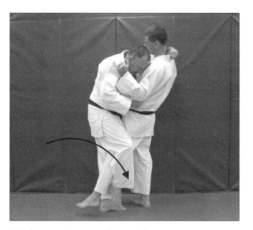

Without releasing forward pressure on your opponent, wrap your right leg behind his left leg and hook it.

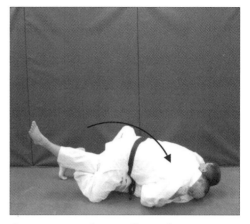

Continuing with your forward momentum, drive your opponent backward and twist toward his left shoulder. Drive your opponent to the ground staying tight and maintaining a dominant position so that you can follow up with groundwork as needed.

Osoto Gake—Drunkle

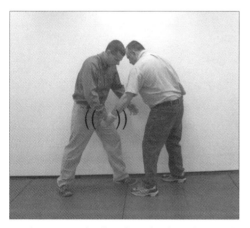

With your right hand grab the adversary's left arm, in this instance, at the wrist. An outside to inside scooping motion with the right hand to capture the adversary's left arm is also acceptable.

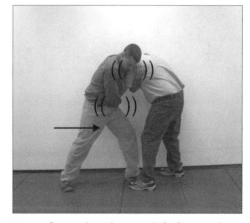

Drive forward with your left foot, seeking the centerline between your adversary's feet. Swing your left arm out into your adversary's left armpit as deep and as far as possible, and simultaneously place your head on his shoulder.

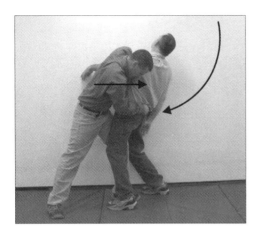

With your left arm, lift high in a circular motion upward and with your right hand grab back center of your adversary's pants, belt, or any available piece of clothing. Grab as close as possible to the base of the spine.

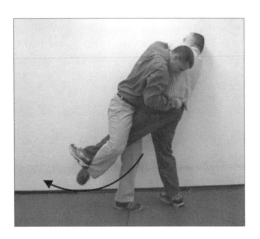

Continue with your forward momentum, reach with your right leg around your adversary's left leg, and then hook, scoop, and lift him into the air.

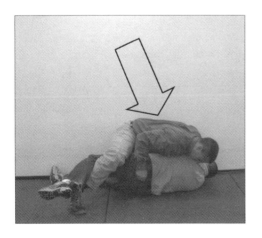

Drive your adversary to the ground, landing on top of him and continuing with the dominant position.

Osoto Gake—Combat

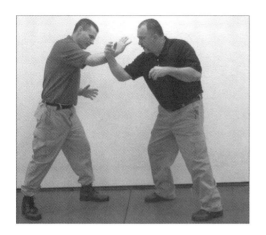

As the attacker reaches or punches with his right hand, intercept his arm with your right arm, making contact with the other guy's arm as soon as possible.

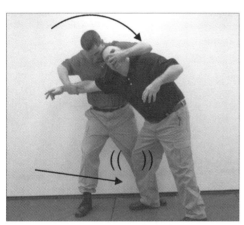

Immediately pivot to the outside. The next three aspects of the movement are important. They must be done simultaneously. With your right hand you are hooking the attacker's right hand, stretching it across your abdomen in an attempt to lock his elbow against your rib cage. Secondly, your left hand comes around the back of the attacker's head, grabbing the chin and pulling his face in the opposite direction of the arm. Thirdly, it's important to use your left knee to drive into your attacker's right knee in an attempt to collapse or compromise it. Although this description breaks these movements into three pieces, it is important that all three be done swiftly and at the same time.

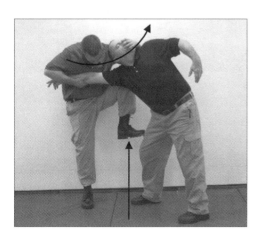

Continuing to hold pressure on the attacker's arm, pull his neck farther while lifting your left foot in preparation to stomp the other guy's right knee.

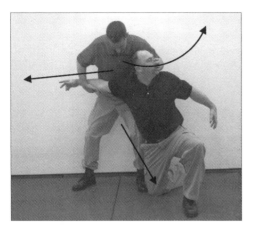

Stomping the attacker's knee into the ground, continue to stand on the knee joint, pinning him.

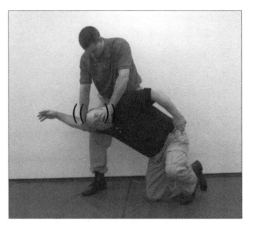

Release the attacker's right hand and put pressure onto the top of his skull, pushing down. With your left hand, lift up in an attempt to wrench the other guy's neck even farther.

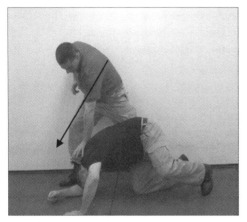

With your left hand, push the attacker's head to the ground.

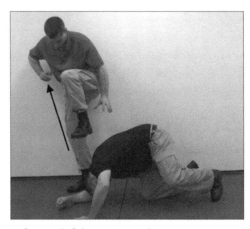

Lift your left leg again with intent to stomp.

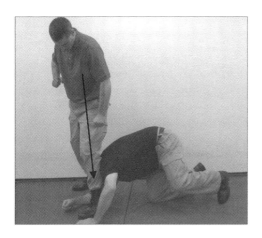

Stomp to the back of the neck. Alternate targets can be the other guy's nearest elbow, or even his spine. Once again, you're stomping on a downed, "helpless" victim. Be sure you can justify this in court.

Head and Arm Drag

The arm drag is, at its essence, a means of pulling your opponent close to employ another technique and/or to get a superior position. The head drag is a gross act of aggression. Simply put, control of the other guy's head is as close as you can come to controlling his entire body without actually enveloping him. Combining these two techniques, especially on a non-grappler, is a swift means of controlling an altercation.

Head and Arm Drag—Competition

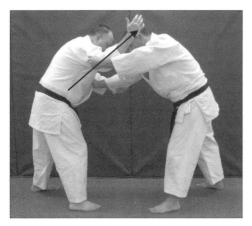

As the opponent steps in with intent to establish his grip, you grab his right sleeve with your left hand and place your right hand on the back of his neck.

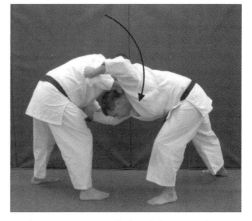

Push your opponent's head downward using your right hand while pulling with your left hand.

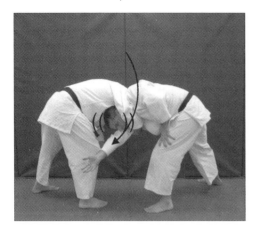

Using your left hand, push the opponent's right arm across his body in front of his face. Keeping your opponent's head in your armpit, bring your right hand from the back of his neck around and across his face and grabbing the back of his right arm (digging your fingertips into his triceps muscles).

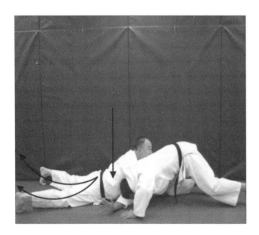

Sprawl, kick your feet back into the air, and drive your belt knot down into the mat. Arch your body as much as you can, placing as much weight on the opponent's head and shoulders as possible.

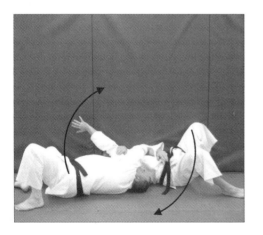

Dropping your left shoulder, begin to roll so that your chest is exposed to the sky, turning your opponent over onto his back.

Head and Arm Drag—Drunkle

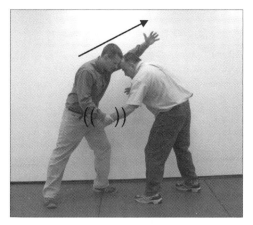

As the adversary steps in with intent to establish his grip, grab his left arm with your right hand and drop your arm with a crashing motion onto the back of his neck.

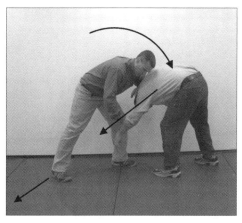

As your forearm lands on the back of the head, pull the adversary's right arm forward and toward the ground while stepping back with your right foot to aid in weight and momentum.

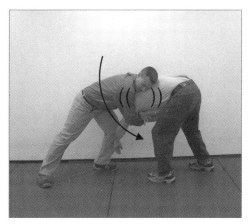

Release your grip on the adversary's arm, strike a blow to the back of his head, and then wrap your left arm around his neck. Tuck your right arm in underneath the other guy's armpit and cinch tightly with intent to obstruct his breathing.

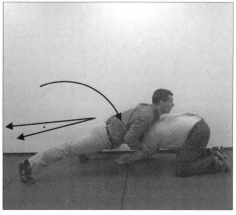

Sprawl, kick your feet back into the air, and drive your belt buckle (or naval if you prefer) onto the ground. Be sure to look upward, creating as much arch in your body as you can so that you place as much weight as possible onto the head and shoulders of your adversary.

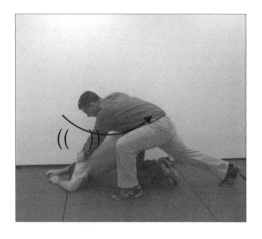

Release your grip, placing both hands on the back of the other guy's neck. Grab any available clothing (or hair) to aid in control if you can. Hold your adversary's face to the ground and pivot your body directly behind him assuming a dominant position.

Head and Arm Drag—Combat

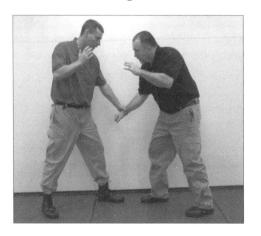

Many options are available, but in this instance we're linking up with a grab to the hand.

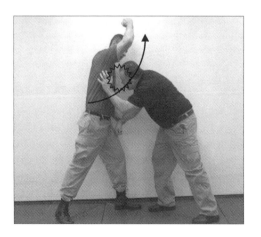

In an explosive motion, use a right rising elbow strike or forearm shiver to strike the attacker's face.

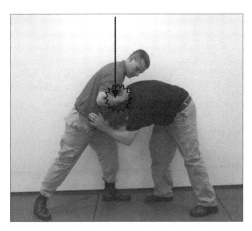

Immediately drop a forearm or hammerfist onto the back of your attacker's neck.

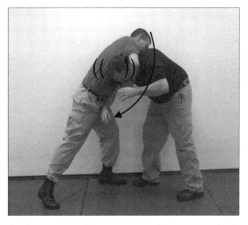

Snake your right arm around your attacker's throat and grab your left hand/arm that has come underneath the other guy's armpit. Apply a choke.

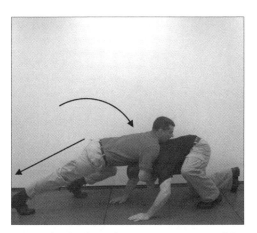

Using the backward momentum created by your right leg, kick out into a sprawl. Stay on your toes. It does not matter if your opponent goes all the way to the ground or stays on his hands and knees (as shown in this picture).

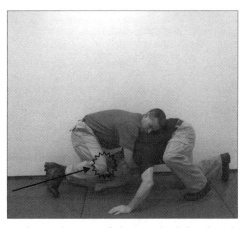

Strike to the top of the attacker's head with your right knee.

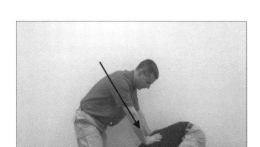

Using both hands between the shoulder blades, shove your attacker face down into the ground. This is similar to a cardiopulmonary respiration (CPR) motion. Use this CPR motion to strike the other guy while aiding you in standing up.

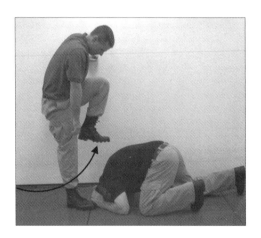

In this instance you use your left foot, but either foot will work. Lift your knee high with intent to stomp.

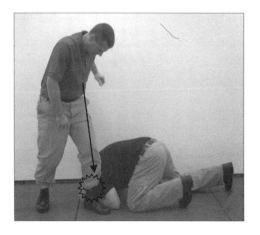

Deliver a stomp to the back of the attacker's neck. Yeah, we've already said this a hundred times, but here it is again: be prepared to justify this in court.

Hammerlock/Front Chancery

The hammerlock/front chancery is a bread-and-butter technique used by wrestlers of all levels and pay scales. The hammerlock/front chancery can also be called a "chicken wing," especially when done from the rear. Regardless of whatever you call it, the purpose of the hammerlock/front chancery is to immobilize the attacker by driving him into the mat or ground, or possibly a wall or other foreign object. The hammerlock/front chancery is done when two opponents are standing and facing each other.

The hammerlock/front chancery immobilizes the other guy's shoulder, locking the highly mobile shoulder joint by forcing it toward the rear of the opponent's body, the area of least mobility. Then the move is completed by forcing the other guy's forearm and elbow upward toward his head, which tightens the shoulder joint even further.

A note on the hammerlock/front chancery: As a general rule, the older the person that is experiencing the lock, the less range of movement he or she will likely have in the shoulder joint. This smaller range means that the lock comes on faster and with less effort. This lack of mobility can also mean faster and more acute injury to the victim. This should be taken into consideration when using the hammerlock/front chancery in situations that most likely do not require incapacitation, such as with social violence scenarios or certain professional roles (e.g., certain security or law enforcement applications).

Hammerlock/Front Chancery—Competition

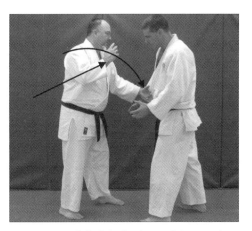

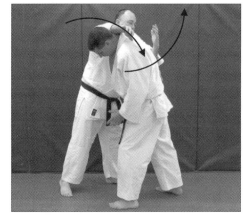

Using your left hand, drop downward to clear the opponent's hands. At the same time reach with your right hand toward the opponent's right shoulder.

Shifting to the right, to the outside of the opponent, grab the back of his neck while scooping upward into the armpit with your left arm.

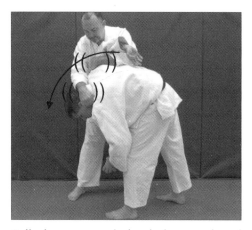

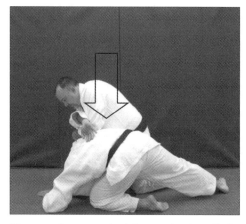

Pull the opponent's head downward and inward toward your body while continuing the outward shift to the opponent's right side. Use your left arm high and on top of the shoulder to lock it and simultaneously create pressure.

Drop to the ground while continuing all the locks, pulls, and motions described in the previous pictures.

Hammerlock/Front Chancery—Drunkle

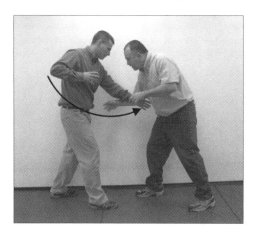

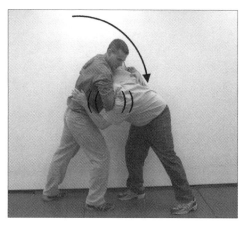

As the adversary moves forward, dive your left hand into the gap between his right arm and right ribs.

Move forward, reach deeply and with an upward scooping motion, placing your left palm on the adversary's back (wrestlers know this as a chicken wing). Keeping your right arm on the same side of the adversary's head, swiftly wrap your arm over the back of his neck. Use your forearm to create pressure on the other guy's throat.

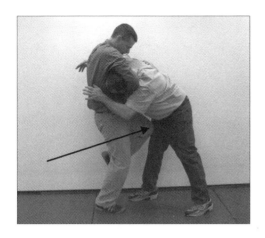

Drive your left knee into the adversary's forward thigh (using either knee is acceptable). The groin and solar plexus are good alternative targets.

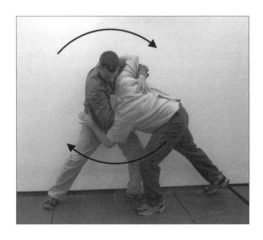

Stepping off to the right side (and in this instance forward) and into your opponent, lift your left arm and assist in rotation with your right arm on the adversary's neck.

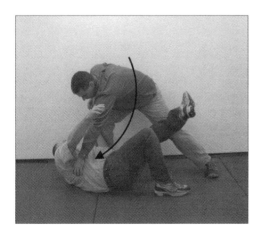

Spin the adversary onto his back while keeping on your feet.

Hammerlock/Front Chancery—Combat

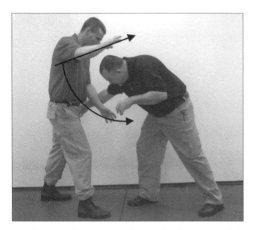

As the attacker moves forward, dive your left hand into the gap between his right arm and right ribs.

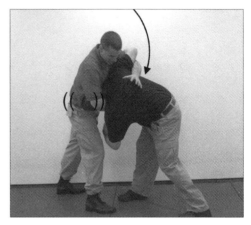

Move forward, reach deeply and with an upward scooping motion, placing your left palm on the attacker's back. Keeping your right arm on the same side of the attacker's head, swiftly wrap your arm over the back of his neck and use your forearm to create pressure on his throat.

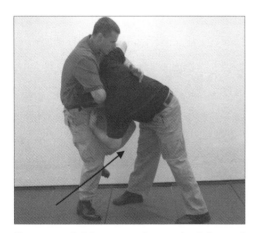

Drive your left knee into the attacker's forward thigh. The groin and solar plexus are good alternative targets.

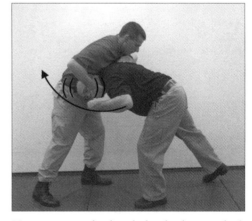

Using your right hand, hook the attacker's chin. Pull swiftly and strongly with intent to wrench his neck.

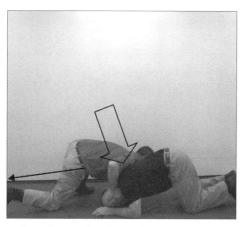

Pulling the attacker forward, drop your weight using your chest in a sprawling motion.

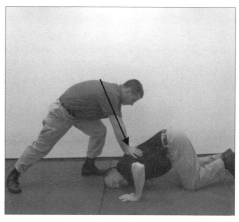

Using your hands placed on the attacker's back, hold him down while using the other guy's body to help you get to your feet.

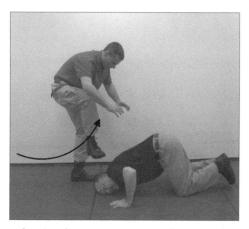

Lift either foot, in this instance the right, with intent to stomp the attacker's head.

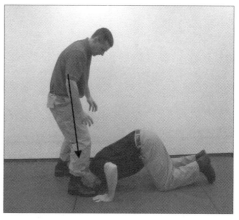

Using your full bodyweight, stomp on the attacker's neck. And, of course, be able to justify why you needed to do this.

Clothesline

The clothesline is a technique that involves using the inside of your extended arm to strike the opponent in the chest, throat, or head. The clothesline can be used in combination with leg sweeps or trips, but also can be effective by itself. The goal of the clothesline is to take the other guy off his feet, doing as much damage as possible in the process.

The clothesline can cause whiplash and neck trauma. The potential for serious injury is so strong that it is banned as a means of tackling a heavily armored (American) football player, in all forms of the game and at all levels. In fact, it carries the highest potential game penalty in yardage assessed (lost), and even includes the possibility of the offending player being ejected from the game, fined, and expelled for several games in the future. In rugby, a high tackle is often referred to as a clothesline too. Regardless of the sport, or the combat application, the clothesline can be brutal and potentially crippling when applied effectively.

Clothesline—Competition

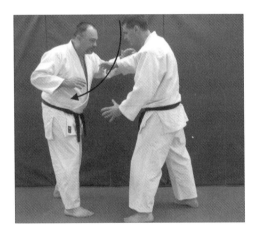

As the opponent comes in to get his grip, use your left hand to swat his right hand down and away, across his body.

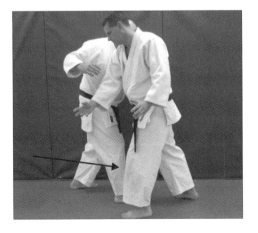

Step forward with your right foot, simultaneously bringing your right hand up with the intent to come across the opponent's throat/chin.

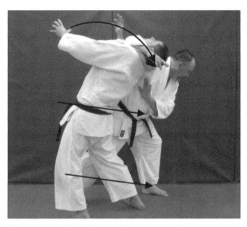

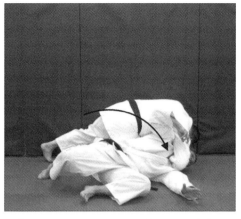

Continue the forward motion by stepping through with your left foot. Poke the opponent's throat/chin with an initial upward motion and then downward, using your upper body's motion to add weight and momentum.

Ride your opponent onto the ground, keeping your leg tightly wrapped around his upper body to assure that you keep your dominant position.

Clothesline—Drunkle

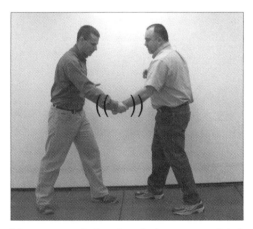

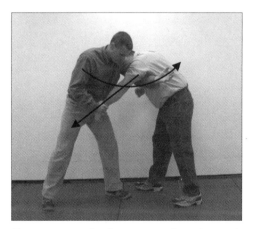

Using your right hand, grab the opponent's left wrist. It is also possible to do this with a slap, moving the other guy's hand/arm across his own centerline to tie him up.

Shoot your right bicep into the adversary's armpit.

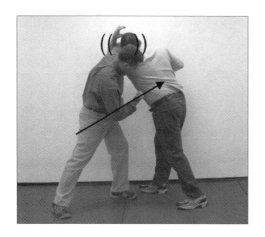

In one swift motion using your left hand as a hook, pull through the opponent's armpit, capturing his triceps. The intent is to pull the adversary high and away, exposing his ribs for a right uppercut to his floating ribs.

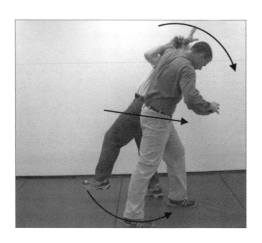

Sweep your left arm into the other guy's throat/chin, lifting upward initially and then sharply downward, using your upper body to add momentum and weight. Simultaneously, step through in order to move behind your opponent.

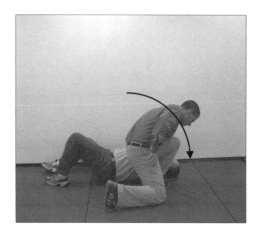

Using your left hand, press your adversary onto the ground. Take a knee beside him with intent to follow up if necessary, either by striking or grappling.

Clothesline—Combat

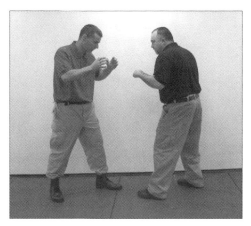

Using your right hand, grab the attacker's left wrist. It is also possible to do this with a slap, moving his hand/arm across his own centerline to tie him up.

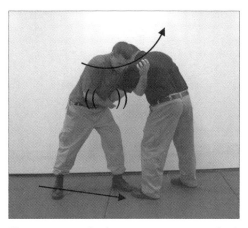

Shoot your right bicep into your attacker's armpit.

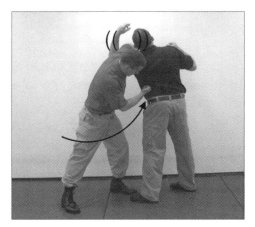

In one swift motion using your left hand as a hook, pull through the opponent's armpit, entangling his triceps. The intent is to pull your opponent high and away, exposing him to an uppercut to his floating ribs.

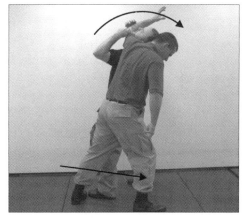

Sweep your left arm into your attacker's throat/chin, lifting upward initially and then sharply downward, using your upper body for momentum and weight. Simultaneously, step through behind your attacker.

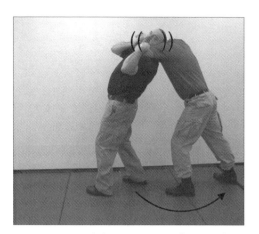

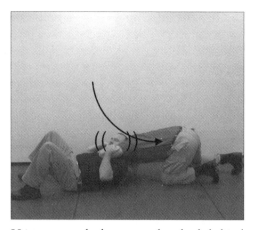

Keeping your left arm across the attacker's throat, reach up with your right hand, grab your own left hand, and apply a "naked" choke while continuing to move backward.

Using a sprawl, shoot your legs back behind you and drop to the ground while applying the choke. Use your shoulder to leverage the attacker's head forward.

Ogoshi

Ogoshi, the major outer throw, is from the original set of throws codified by the founder of judo, Jigoro Kano. *Ogoshi* was not created by Kano, however. In fact, it probably ranks high in the pantheon of "the first technique a man ever used to attack another man," right up there with hitting with a clenched fist or whacking the other guy with a stick. The reason for its high ranking is its simplicity and effectiveness.

One reason for the effectiveness of this technique is that it involves lifting the opponent off the ground. Once the attacker is off the ground, not linked to the earth, he has no traction, little friction, and only a small control of his body. This lack of control places you at an enormous advantage and allows you to slam your opponent into the ground, in effect using the ground as a striking weapon. Unlike a soft judo or wrestling mat, the ground can pack one heck of a wallop, particularly when it's uneven, rock strewn, or littered with debris.

Ogoshi—Competition

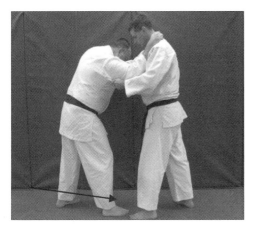

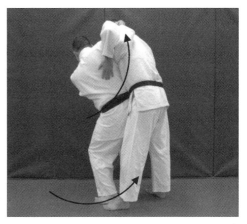

Using a regular competitive judo grip, right hand on collar and left hand on the opponent's right elbow, step forward with your right foot.

Turn 180 degrees, pulling with your left arm and lifting with your right hand. Leave no space between you and your opponent. Place your waist underneath your opponent's waist. This assures that your center of gravity is lower, displacing your opponent's weight and center of balance.

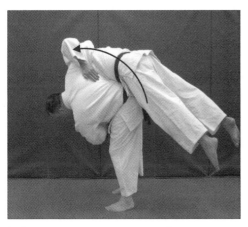

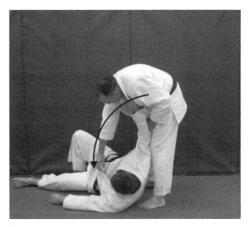

Lift your opponent onto your hip.

Drop your opponent to the ground over your waist. Remain standing.

Ogoshi—Drunkle

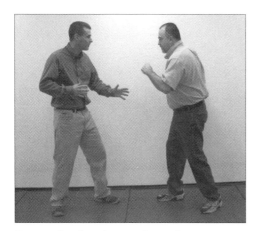

Prepare for the adversary's attack.

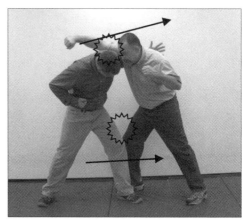

As the adversary throws a right hook (obviously this can be done to either side), dive forward with intent to strike with a head butt. Use your left knee to check the other guy's right knee. NOTE: For a head butt, turn away, protecting the face.

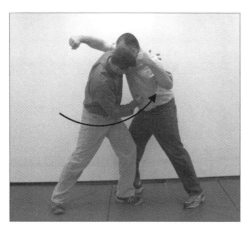

Drive an uppercut into the adversary's solar plexus.

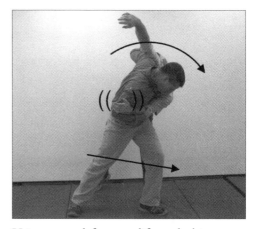

Using your left arm, lift and drive your adversary's right arm upward and into his face. Pull the adversary's left arm across your chest while stepping forward with your left leg, driving the other guy backward.

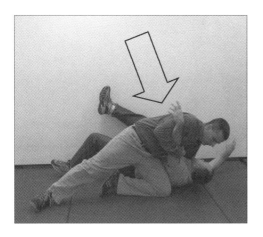

Landing on your opponent, pin him to the ground with your bodyweight. Don't hang out on the ground unless you have a need to secure the adversary and have determined that it is safe to do so.

Ogoshi—Combat

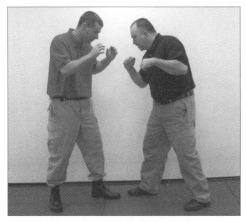

Prepare for the attack.

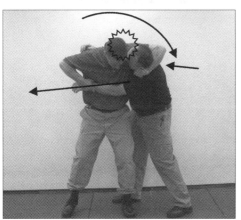

As the attacker leads with his left hand (however a right does not change your response), grab his left arm and pull while swinging your left arm around the back of the other guy's head. Pull his head toward your head to set up a head butt strike.

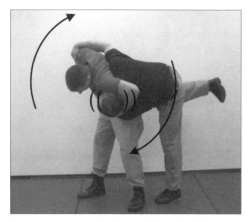

Twist your attacker by pulling his left arm, using his head as a fulcrum.

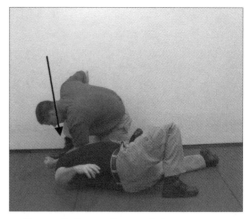

Pull your left arm free and then using your bodyweight, crush your forearm into the attacker's neck.

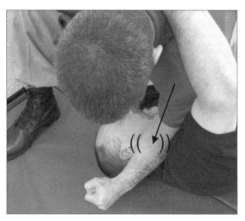

Here is a close up of forearm/elbow to neck, demonstrating the proper positioning.

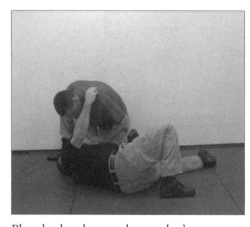

Place both palms on the attacker's sternum.

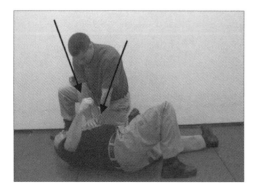

With your bodyweight, drive both palms into the chest with intent to separate, crack, or break the attacker's ribs. This technique can be made to look inadvertent, even on closed circuit or cellphone video if you do it properly, not that we'd suggest that or anything...

Uchi Mata

Uchi mata is an inner thigh throw. It is used to put the other guy on the ground by controlling and lifting his center of gravity (hips) with your upper, inner thigh. The classification of *uchi mata* varies as it is sometimes described as a leg throw and sometimes referred to as a hip throw. It doesn't really matter; we believe that the key is to highlight the action a practitioner must use for success.

Used in all throwing arts, including judo, *jujitsu*, and *sumo*, it can be performed with or without a uniform (some throws rely on the other guy's uniform which is no big deal in competition, but sometimes a real bugger on the street if you face an adversary who is shirtless or wearing lightweight clothing). Similar to other lifting throws, its success is based on the separation of the attacker from the ground. Follow-up usually means landing on the other guy. This places you in a dominant position and allows for a quick follow-up with pins, locks, chokes, or blows. *Uchi mata* is one of the most popular throws in judo competition and is used across weight classes.

Uchi Mata—Competition

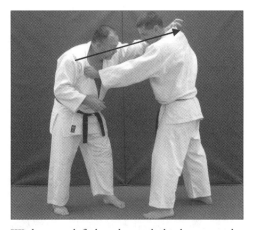 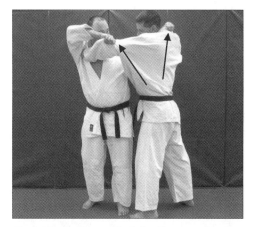

With your left hand, reach high on to the opponent's collar and grip it in preparation for the throw.

Grab the opponent's left elbow with your right hand. Lift both hands high, simultaneously pulling the opponent in toward yourself.

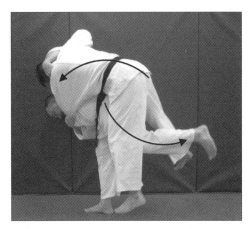

Lifting your opponent onto your hip, shoot your left leg between your opponent's legs, and then lift his inner right thigh to keep him balanced on your hip.

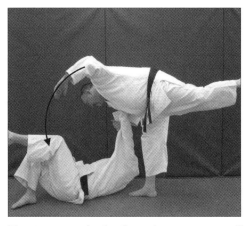

Twisting your body, fling the opponent off your hip and onto the ground.

Uchi Mata—Drunkle

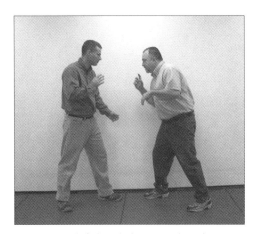

Drop your left hand downward with intent to invite a right-hand strike from your adversary.

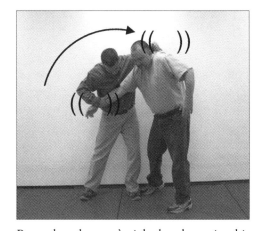

Parry the adversary's right hand, passing his hand and reaching the back of his neck as you simultaneously step and grab his right hand (or forearm) with your right hand.

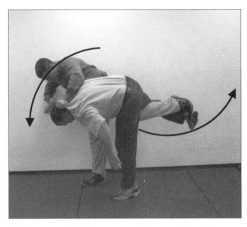

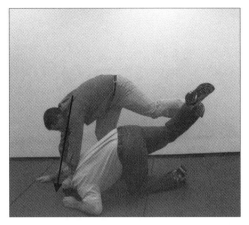

Lift your left leg into the inside of your adversary's right leg and drive his head forward. Continue to hold on to the opponent's right arm (an over-the-top hook and pin also works). In this example, the back collar of the shirt is grabbed and used to force the head forward, but cupping the back of the other guy's head with an open palm is also an option.

Force the adversary forward and off your leg, driving his face onto the ground.

Uchi Mata—Combat

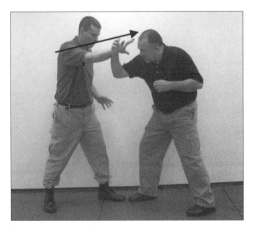

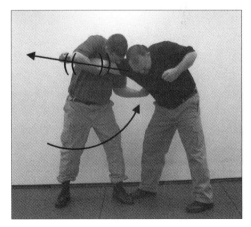

Using your right hand, strike to the other guy's face in order to draw a right block from the attacker.

Grab the attacker's right arm, pulling and striking to his ribs with an uppercut.

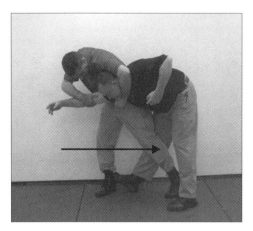

Reach over the top and behind the attacker's head, and grab his chin. Then, using your left leg, kick backward into the attacker's right leg with intent to hyperextend his knee (optimally) or get the other guy to lift his leg in order to avoid your strike.

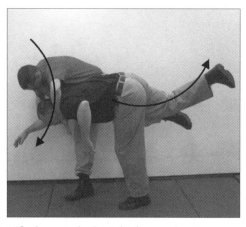

Lift the attacker's right leg, and using your left arm, simultaneously drive his face forward and to the ground.

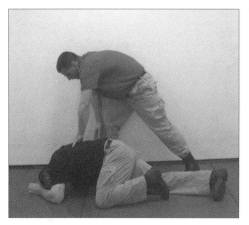

Use your left hand to push/hold the attacker down.

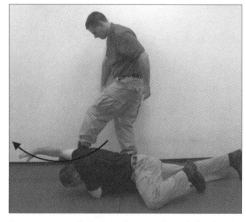

Swing your left leg forward and kick the attacker's right arm.

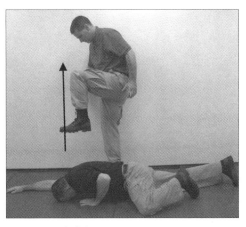

Raise your left leg to stomp.

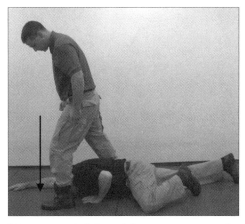

Using your left leg, deliver a stomp to the head or neck of your attacker. And, as always, be sure you can justify this if it goes to court.

Sukui Nage

Wrestlers would call *sukui nage*, or scooping throw, a double leg take down. *Sukui nage* is used most commonly as a counter to an aggressive high attack and not necessarily a primary technique. However, with proper timing and a degree of skillfulness, *sukui nage* can be employed as an aggressive primary attack.

Sukui Nage—Competition

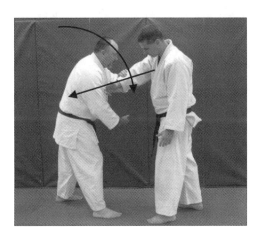

Using your left arm, grab the opponent's right arm. Your right arm is coming upward with intent to subsequently transfer the opponent's right hand to your own right hand.

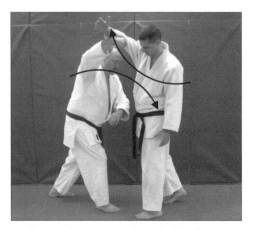

Exchange the opponent's right hand to your right hand and lift it high as you bring your left shoulder forward with intent to drive your left arm across the opponent's body.

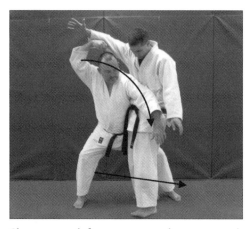

Shoot your left arm across the opponent's abdomen while stepping forward behind his right leg into a low, wide stance.

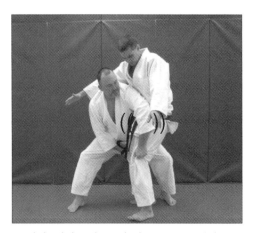

With both hands, grab the opponent's knees (grabbing the *gi* pants or scooping behind the knees, whichever works).

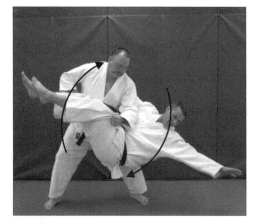

Simultaneously, drive your left shoulder into the opponent's chest and lift with both hands, pulling the legs out from underneath the opponent.

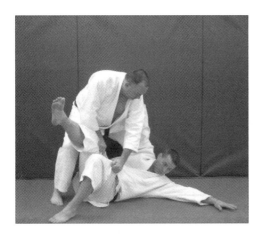

As the opponent lands on the ground, keep on your feet.

Sukui Nage—Drunkle

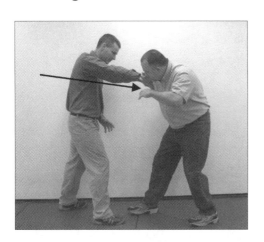

Reach out with your right hand and seize the adversary's right wrist or arm.

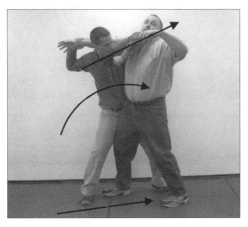

With your left leg, step behind the adversary's right leg. Simultaneously, slip under the adversary's arm to gain position so you can hit the other guy's chin with your left elbow.

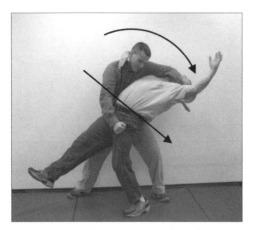

Sweep your left arm across the adversary's face and bend him backward over your left thigh. Let go of your adversary's right arm, dropping it to his waist to hold him in position.

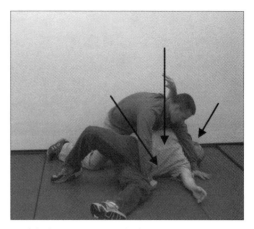

Hold the adversary down with your chest. Create pressure by pulling backward across his throat and groin while driving your left knee into the adversary's back to create three points of pressure.

Sukui Nage—Combat

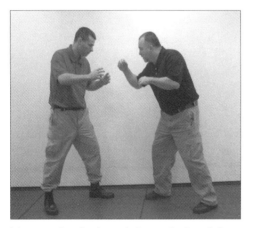

The attacker leads with his right hand for a possible punch or grab.

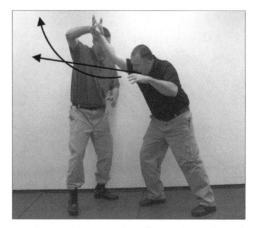

As the attacker reaches forward, grab and guide his arm upward while pulling.

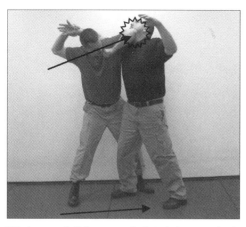

With your left leg, step behind the attacker's right leg, simultaneously slipping under the other guy's arm to gain position so that you can hit his chin with your left elbow.

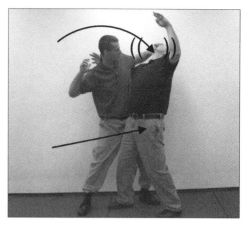

Use your body to push into your attacker, continuing to drive your elbow into his throat/face.

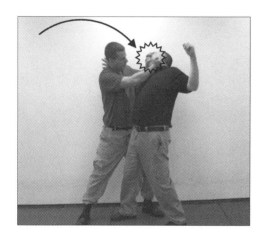

Pull your left arm across the face of the attacker, using a tiger claw. Strike with a hammerfist to the exposed side of the throat, aiming for the carotid artery.

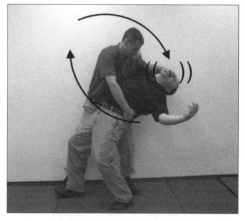

Keeping your left hand in a claw, drive his face backward while using your right hand to pull and lock his back (picking the attacker's left leg is an alternative to pulling at the waist).

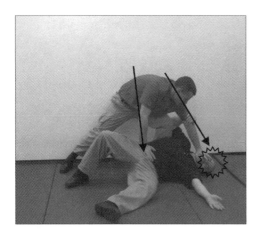

Slip your right hand to the attacker's stomach, and push the left and right hands downward with the intent to slam the other guy's head into the ground.

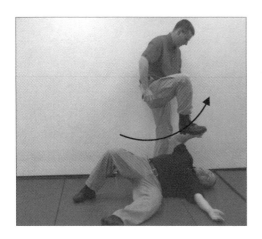

Lift your right leg up in a stepping motion in preparation to stomp.

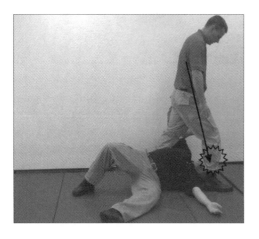

Stomp the attacker's face/neck. And, of course, be able to justify your actions.

Hammerlock

The hammerlock is a classic tool of law enforcement, used when detaining a person and facilitating the application of handcuffs. The suspect's hand is put behind his back, the back of his hand touching his spine. This position locks the suspect's shoulder reducing his range of motion. No matter how flexible, even the most mobile joint can be taken out of play when locked properly. Furthermore, the hammerlock allows for a high level of control, if necessary, forcing the suspect's hand upward along the spine, toward the neck, creating pressure and pain in the same shoulder and more than likely forcing him onto his toes in an effort to gain relief from the pain. Not all threats actually feel pain, so this does not work on everyone. Often, an officer will bend the wrist of the hand secured behind the suspect—think of the fingers pointing out of the suspect's back like the dorsal fin on a fish. This hand position creates three points of stress: the wrist, the elbow, and the shoulder, for a 3:1 ratio of control, three joints controlled with one hand.

Hammerlock—Competition

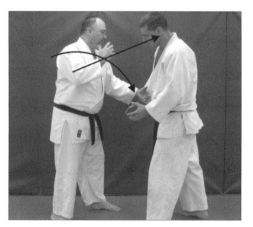

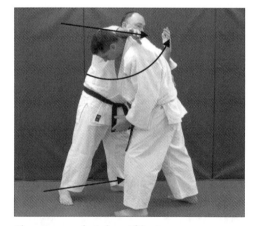

As the opponent reaches toward you, knock down his right hand with your left hand, using a downward sweeping motion.

Shoot your hand swiftly into your opponent's armpit as if doing a bicep curl. At the same time, shift your body to the outside by shuffling forward with your left foot. With your right hand, reach over your opponent's right shoulder, placing your hand on the back of his head.

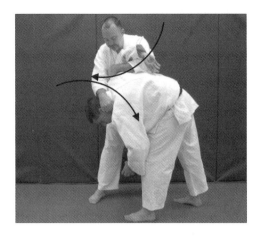

Place your left hand on the back of your opponent's shoulder joint, pushing down with your left hand while lifting slightly with your left elbow. Use your right hand to force your opponent's head downward in conjunction with the pressure placed on his right shoulder.

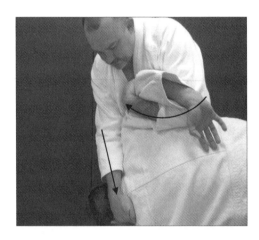

Close-up of hammerlock, pushing downward on opponent's neck.

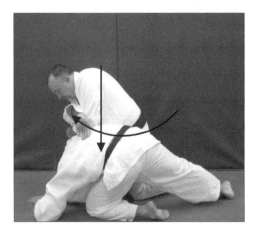

As your opponent is forced onto the ground, go down with him.

Hammerlock—Drunkle

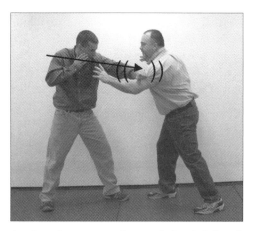

As the adversary reaches with his left hand, reach out with your left hand and grab his shoulder to jam his attack.

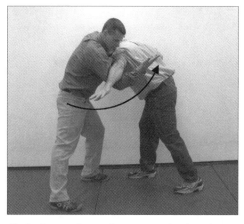

Shift forward. With your right hand, use a scooping motion to go underneath the adversary's left arm. It is important to get chest to chest, as close as possible at this point, to avoid being hit by a strong right hand counterpunch.

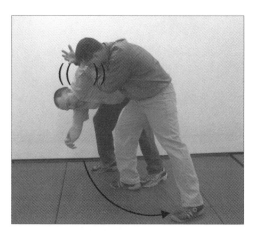

Stepping forward with your right foot, get as close to your adversary's left foot as you can without actually stepping on his foot. Swing to the outside with your left foot, holding the other guy's shoulder joint tightly and apply a downward, sustaining pressure.

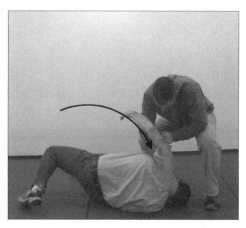

Drop into a horse stance, forcing your adversary's shoulder to the ground.

Hammerlock—Combat

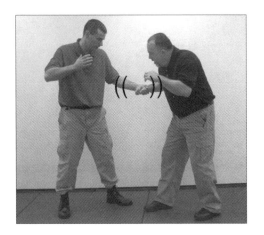

Reach out with your left hand, grabbing your attacker's wrist. It is also possible to use your left hand and outward block while diving inward instead, but in this instance control of the wrist is important.

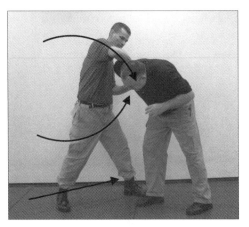

Shifting forward with the left foot, move to the outside line of your attacker. Maneuvering his shoulder at your sternum, reach over the top of the attacker's shoulder with your right hand. The intent of your right hand is to place as much downward pressure on the other guy's elbow as possible.

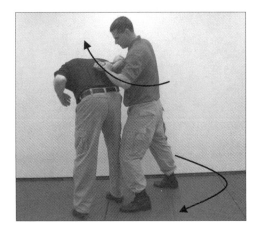

Continue this spinning motion by moving your right foot in a swinging arc behind you. It is important at this point that maximum pressure is placed on the attacker's shoulder so that he cannot escape. This pressure is created by forcing the other guy's left hand up the line of his spine while simultaneously pushing his elbow downward.

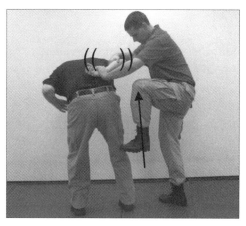

Lift your right foot with intent to strike the back of your attacker's right knee. Using your left leg frees up your right foot for a follow-up strike.

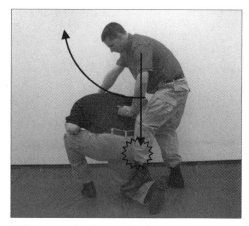

Lift your right foot with the intent to stomp to the other guy's head, neck, or ribs.

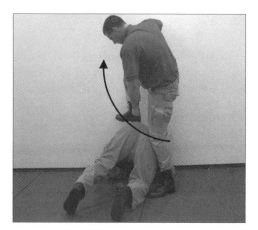

Lift knee with intent to stomp again.

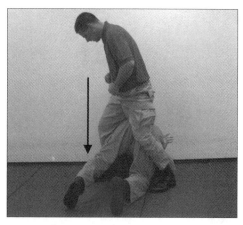

Stomp downward, using the heel of your boot for maximum effect. And, of course, be able to justify your actions.

Ude Hishigi Waki Gatame

A combination of an arm lock using the armpit, these two techniques are mixed and matched with other pins and locks to force an opponent to submit. In combat, they can be used to destroy the elbow joint separating the humerus from the radius and ulna. This combination also creates a higher level of safety for defending against an attack because it places the other guy in a poor position to continue his assault, while you are turning your vulnerable areas away from the threat. Powerfully applied, the attack is crippling since it places your entire body against the attacker's elbow joint, combines gravity, leverage, and percussive force resulting in a powerful concoction, a perfect storm of advantage and disadvantage.

Ude Hishigi Waki Gatame—Competition

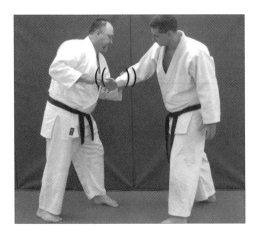

With your left hand, grab your opponent's right sleeve.

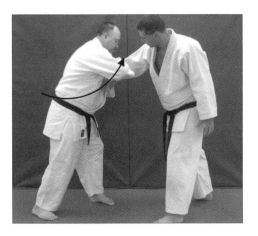

Reach up and grab the same arm you just captured with your right hand.

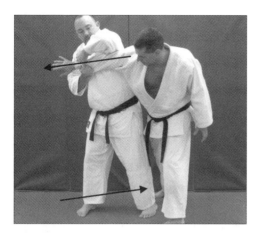

Using your two hands as the pivot point, twist your body around the arm placing pressure on the opponent's elbow. Shuffle your left foot in between your opponent's legs.

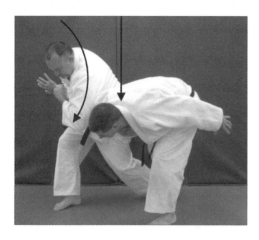

Pinch your opponent's right triceps tightly into your armpit while pulling his wrist upward. Twist away from your opponent to add momentum while intensifying the lock.

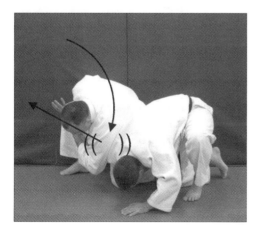

Continue to leverage your opponent onto the ground, pulling his arm and driving downward with your armpit.

Ude Hishigi Waki Gatame—Drunkle

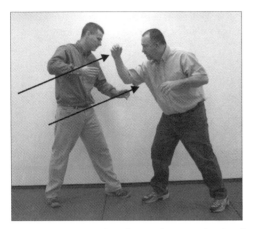

As adversary reaches forward, move both of your hands to meet his attack and slip to the outside of his right arm.

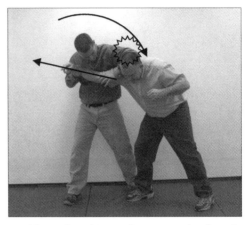

Grabbing the adversary's wrist, strike the side of his face with your left elbow.

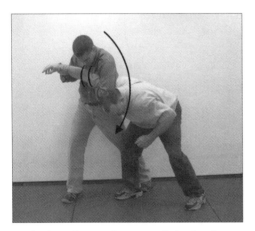

Grab the adversary's arm with both of your hands. Pinch his triceps tightly between your arm and ribcage.

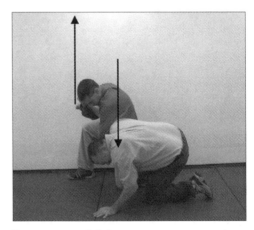

Drop to your left knee, using your armpit to create downward pressure while simultaneously lifting the other guy's wrist upward and away from your center.

Ude Hishigi Waki Gatame—Combat

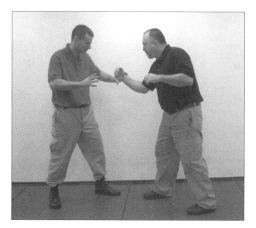

With your left hand, grab the attacker's right arm.

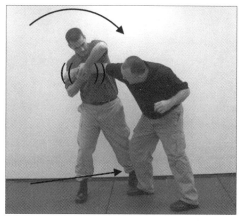

Reach up and grab the same arm with your right hand. Use your ribcage as a fulcrum to lock the attacker's elbow.

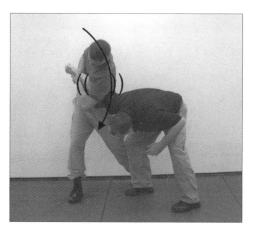

Using both your hands as a pivot point, twist your body around the attacker's arm placing pressure on his elbow. Shuffle your left foot to the outside of the attacker's body.

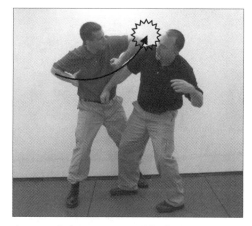

As you feel pressure, suddenly reverse your direction swinging back into the attacker's face with your left elbow.

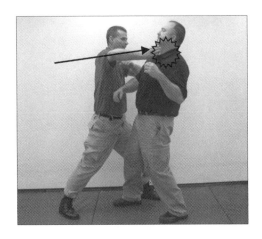

Deliver a right open palm strike to throat of the attacker.

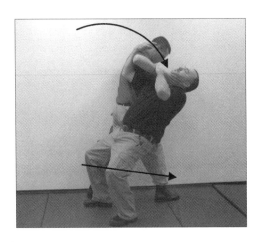

With your right leg, step behind the attacker and drive his head to the ground.

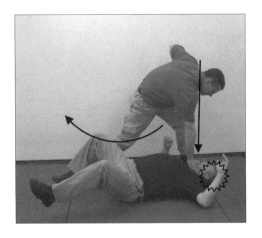

Continuing this motion, strike attacker's throat with your right hand. As always, be justified.

Whizzer

An aggressive technique in both attacking and countering, the whizzer is in the top drawer of most any wrestler's metaphorical toolbox of techniques. The whizzer is used to move the adversary's body, using his shoulder as the root of the action. By locking up the other guy's arm at the top of his triceps and into the armpit, the technique can cinch a tight grip close his body or be used as a percussive strike. This cinching allows you to move the adversary's body, often forward and down, making it difficult for the other guy to immediately counter. It forces the other guy into at least one defensive move in an attempt to deal with the pressure applied to his armpit and shoulder. The whizzer as a strike is violent and jarring, often used to break or cut a take down, and gain separation.

Whizzer—Competition

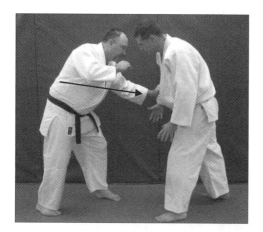

Reach out and grab the opponent's wrist.

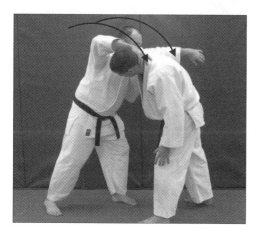

As the opponent reacts to your grab, put your right hand on the back of his head and reach over the top of his right arm.

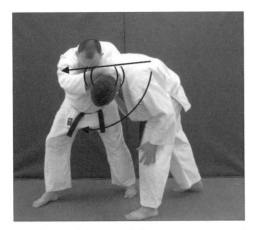

Cinch your left arm tightly as it wraps around the opponent's right arm, high at the armpit. Simultaneously, put downward pressure on the back of his neck.

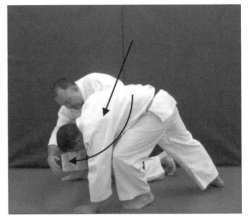

Drop to a knee to make your opponent bear your full bodyweight, while twisting forward and driving him forward.

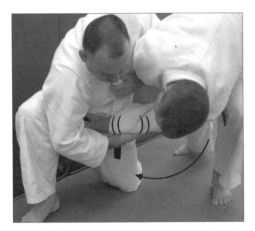

Once you release the opponent's head with your right hand, reach across and grab the opponent's left arm that he is using to hold himself up, and scoop the arm toward yourself.

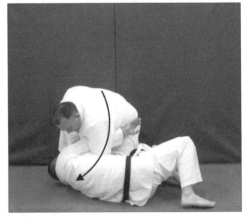

Drive your left shoulder forward as you pull to turn your opponent onto his back.

Whizzer—Drunkle

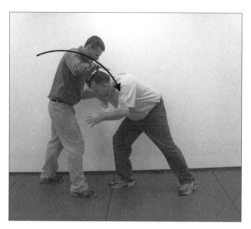

As the adversary reaches in for a grab or tackle, shoot your left hand downward in front of his shoulder to block the attempt. Place your right hand on top of the other guy's head or neck.

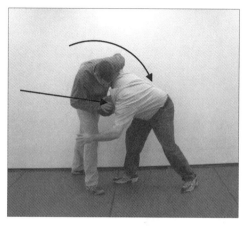

Shove the adversary's head downward while lifting your left arm and pulling the other guy's right armpit, to twist him and disrupt his balance.

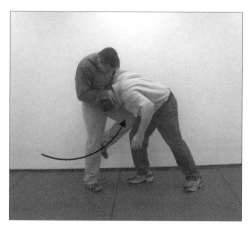

Strike upward with your left knee into the adversary's face or solar plexus.

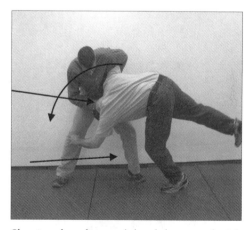

Shoving the adversary's head downward with your right hand while lifting his armpit with your left, step with your left leg to the side to unbalance the other guy.

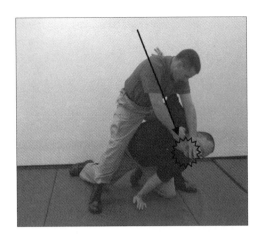

After the adversary lands, step over his head and block his neck, pinning him in place

Whizzer—Combat

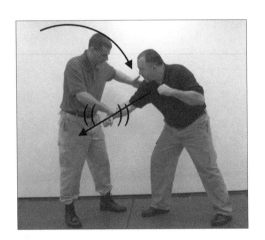

As the attacker reaches forward, meet his leading arm and reach behind, seeking his armpit.

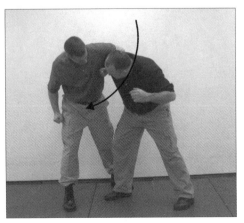

Wrap your arm around the attacker's armpit and twist forward with your left arm to lever his shoulders away. This should avoid any potential left strike.

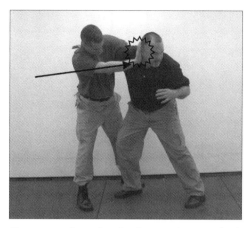

Shoot a right palm heel into the attacker's face to continue to keep any follow-on strike from hitting you.

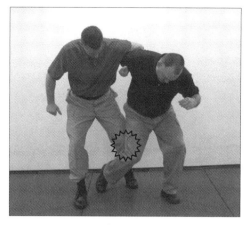

Drive your left knee forward to buckle the attacker's left knee.

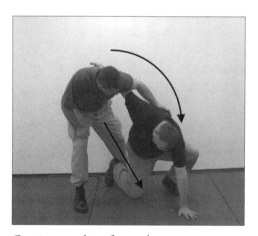

Continue to drive forward.

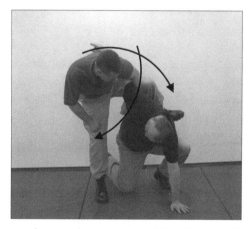

As the attacker stops his fall with his left hand, step over his back while maintaining the armlock.

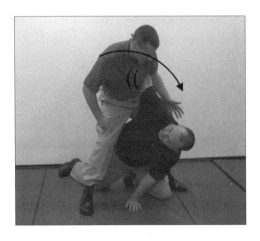

As the attacker begins to turn toward to you to relieve the pressure on his shoulder, continue to drive forward.

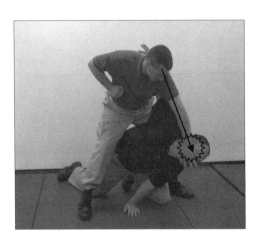

Pop him in the face with a left palm heel strike.

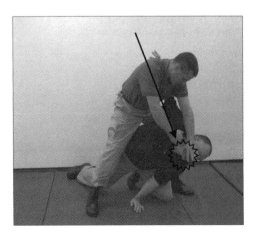

Strike to the neck or jaw with a right straight punch to finish off your attacker.

Conclusion

Ground fighting is an essential component of the martial curriculum. While grappling practitioners are comfortable working in this area, many become overly focused on the sporting aspects, so much so that drunkle and combative applications are overlooked. It's hard to escape from a bad guy if you're working to get him in a lock or hold. And his friends might just decide to kick your head in while you're rolling around on the ground. Conversely, strikers tend to avoid the ground like the plague. The challenge is that oftentimes it's the other guy who forces you to go there. Strikers with no ground game tend to fare poorly when they fall down.

In this book, we provided several examples showing how a single technique can easily be adapted to meet all three types of challenges you may have to deal with. While we have covered a representative sampling, in reality we have barely scratched the surface of everything that's out there. Now it's your turn. Take a look at the applications you like to use, evaluate them, and practice all three variations so that you can readily shift gears as the tactical situation dictates.

Glossary

akharas. Gymnasium or training hall.

bunkai. Fighting application.

bunkai oyo. Standard application (interpretation).

battuere. To beat.

bicallis. Footpath.

bo. Fighting staff.

bökh. Mongolian wrestling.

dojo. Training hall.

drunkle. A combination of the words "drunk" and "uncle," referring to situations in which you need to control a person without severely injuring him.

gastrizein. Straight kick with the bottom of the foot, heal, to the stomach or lower abdomen.

Genghis Khan. Founded the Mongol Empire. Reigned 1206–1227 BCE. At the height of its power, this empire spanned from the Black Sea to the Korean peninsula.

ghee. Clarified butter.

gi. Traditional practice uniform of Okinawan and Japanese martial arts.

Gort. A padded suit, used for full contact sparring and scenario training. This term comes from the 1951 movie *The Day the Earth Stood Still* because it looks a lot like the robot featured in that film.

guru. Teacher.

hajime. "Begin," the command that starts a judo match.

hiji ate. Elbow strike.

hojo undo. Training using traditional implements that strengthen a *karateka*, similar to modern weight training.

joris. Bowling pins.

judoka. Judo practitioners.

karateka. Karate practitioner.

kata. Forms ("formal exercise").

klimax. Ladder (more specifically the final rung of a ladder or climax of a *pankration* bout).

ko uchi gari. Small, inner reaping throw.

kobudo. A martial art based on using farm implements and "found" tools as weapons

kobudoka. Practitioner of *kobudo*.

koryu. Japanese battlefield martial arts (typically pre-Meiji Restoration era).

kushti. Indian wrestling.

macto. Fighting (also to magnify, glorify, honor, slay, punish, or afflict).

macto bicallis. The fighting way.

makiwara. Striking post.

muay Thai. Is Thailand's national sport. Similar to boxing, *muay Thai* practitioners use boxing gloves and boxing strikes. This sport is also famous for powerful leg kicks and knee strikes.

ne-waza. Groundwork (grappling techniques)

naadam. "Play," a *bökh* sporting event.

nals. Stone weights.

osoto gake. Major outer hooking throw.

osoto gari. Major outer reaping throw.

ogoshi. Major outer throw.

pankration. An ancient martial art (and early Olympic sport) reportedly developed by Hercules.

sukui nage. Scooping throw.

sumtola. Barbells.

tatami. Straw-filled mats traditionally used in judo.

Theodosius I. Roman Emperor 379–395 BCE also known as Theodosius the Great.

uchi komi. A traditional skill-building exercise for *judoka*.

uchi mata. Inner thigh throw.

ude hishigi waki gatame. Traditional judo arm lock.

vseobuch. Russian abbreviation for general military training.

Xerxes. Xerxes I, Persian king, reigned 485–465 BCE.

Bibliography

Books

Adams, Neil. *Armlocks (Judo Masterclass Techniques)* 2nd ed. London, England: Ippon Books Limited, 1989.

Arvanitis, Jim. *Pankration: The Traditional Greek Combat Sport and Modern Martial Art.* Boulder: Paladin Press, 2003.

Burns, Farmer. *Lessons in Wrestling and Physical Culture.* Farmer Burns School of Wrestling, 1913.

Chapman, Mike. *Gotch: An American Hero.* Culture House Books, 1999.

Georgiou, Andreas V. *Pankration: An Olympic Sport* (Volume 1). Philadelphia: Xlibris Corporation, 2005.

Hackenschmidt, George. *The Way to Live.* CreateSpace, 2011.

Dempsey, Jack and Jack Cuddy. Championship Fighting: Explosive Punching and Aggressive Defense. Centerline Press 1983 (original edition was printed in 1950 in NY by Prentice Hall).

Kano, Jigoro. *Kodokan Judo.* New York: Kodansha International/USA. 1986.

Kashiwazaki, Katsuhiko. *Osaekomi (Judo Masterclass Techniques).* London:Ippon Books Limited, 1997.

LaBell, Gene. *Grappling Master: Combat For Street Defense and Competition.* Los Angeles: Pro-Action Publishing, 1992.

Matsushita, Saburo and Warwick Stevens, *Contest Judo: Ten Decisive Throws.*College Station, TX: Ippon Books, USA, 1994.

Mysnyk, Mark, MD, Barry Davis, and Brooks Simpson, *Winning Wrestling Moves.* Champagne, IL: Human Kinetics, 1994.

Sugai, Hitoshi. *Uchimata (Judo Masterclass Techniques).* London: Ippon Books Limited, 1992.

Websites

Amateur Pankration League http://www.fightleague.org/

Ancient Olympics http://ancientolympics.arts.kuleuven.be/eng/TP001EN.html

Cultural China http://www.cultural china.com/chinaWH/html/en/11Kaleidoscope302.html

Encyclopedia Britannica http://www.britannica.com/EBchecked/topic/389419/Mongolian-wrestling

Historical Pankration Project http://historical-pankration.com/article-1.html

International Federation of Pankration http://www.pankration.gr/index.htm

Wikipedia http://en.wikipedia.org/wiki/Mongolian_wrestling

Television

Hitman Hart: Wrestling with Shadows, 1998 TV Movie

Index

About the Authors

Kris Wilder

Kris Wilder is the head instructor and owner of West Seattle Karate Academy. Kris started practicing the martial arts at the age of fifteen. Over the years, he has earned black belt rankings in three styles, *Goju Ryu* karate (5th *dan*), *tae kwon d*o (2nd *dan*), and judo (1st *dan*), in which he has competed in senior national and international tournaments.

He has had the opportunity to train under skilled instructors, including Olympic athletes, state champions, national champions, and gifted martial artists who take their lineage directly from the founders of their systems. Kris has trained across the United States and Okinawa. Kris teaches seminars worldwide. Kris also serves as a National Representative for the University of New Mexico's Institute of Traditional Martial Arts.

Kris is the author of *The Way of Sanchin Kata*, *The Way of Martial Arts for Kids*, and *Lessons from the Dojo Floor* and co-author (with Lawrence Kane) of *The Way of Kata*, *The Way to Black Belt*, *How to Win a Fight*, and *The Little Black Book of Violence*. He also stars in two DVDs, *121 Killer Appz! Fighting Applications from Goju Ryu Karate*, and *Sanchin Kata: Three Battles Karate Kata*. He co-hosts a podcast with Lawrence Kane at www.martial-secrets.com. Kris lives in Seattle, Washington with his son Jackson.

Lawrence A. Kane

Lawrence is the author of *Surviving Armed Assaults*, *Martial Arts Instruction*, and *Blinded by the Night*; co-author (with Kris Wilder) of *The Way of Kata*, *The Way to Black Belt*, *How to Win a Fight*, and *The Little Black Book of Violence;* and co-author (with Rory Miller) of *Scaling Force*. A founding technical consultant to University of New Mexico's Institute of Traditional Martial Arts, he also has written numerous articles on martial arts, self-defense, and related topics for prestigious publications such as the *International Ryukyu Karate-jutsu Research Society Journal, Jissen, Fighting Arts, and Traditional Karate* magazine. His work has also been featured in *Fighter's Fact Book 2: The Street* by Loren Christensen, and *Wicked Wisdom: Explorations into the Dark Side* by Bohdi Sanders and Shawn Kovacich.

Since 1970, he has studied and taught traditional Asian martial arts, medieval European combat, and modern close-quarter weapon techniques. He co-hosts a podcast with Kris Wilder at www.martial-secrets.com. Working stadium security part-time, he has been involved in hundreds of violent altercations, but gets paid to watch football. To cover the bills, he develops sourcing strategies for an aerospace company where he gets to play with billions of dollars of other people's money and make really important decisions. Lawrence lives in Seattle, Washington with his son Joey and wife Julie.

Erik McCray

"Erik McCray is one of the best martial artists we know, humble, pleasant, easy to be around and flat out spooky dangerous when the switch is flipped."

A steel worker by trade, Erik has spent his life training in the martial arts. As a child, he learned basic fighting techniques from his father, a smoke jumper. From there Erik moved into high school wrestling, competitive judo, *jujitsu*, *kung-fu*, and boxing. He also has served as a boxing coach and as a martial arts instructor. Erik lives in Seattle with his wife and two children.

BOOKS FROM YMAA

BOOKS FROM YMAA (continued)

TRADITIONAL TAEKWONDO	B0665
WAY OF KATA	B0584
WAY OF KENDO AND KENJITSU	B0029
WAY OF SANCHIN KATA	B0845
WAY TO BLACK BELT	B0852
WESTERN HERBS FOR MARTIAL ARTISTS	B1972
WILD GOOSE QIGONG	B787
WOMAN'S QIGONG GUIDE	B833
XINGYIQUAN, 2ND ED.	B416

DVDS FROM YMAA

ADVANCED PRACTICAL CHIN NA IN-DEPTH	D1224
ANALYSIS OF SHAOLIN CHIN NA	D0231
BAGUAZHANG—EMEI BAGUAZHANG	D0649
CHEN STYLE TAIJIQUAN	D0819
CHIN NA IN-DEPTH COURSES 1—4	D602
CHIN NA IN-DEPTH COURSES 5—8	D610
CHIN NA IN-DEPTH COURSES 9—12	D629
EIGHT SIMPLE QIGONG EXERCISES FOR HEALTH	D0037
ESSENCE OF TAIJI QIGONG	D0215
FACING VIOLENCE—7 THINGS A MARTIAL ARTIST MUST KNOW	D2283
FIVE ANIMAL SPORTS	D1106
KNIFE DEFENSE—TRADITIONAL TECHNIQUES AGAINST A DAGGER	D1156
KUNG FU BODY CONDITIONING 1	D2085
KUNG FU BODY CONDITIONING 2	D2290
KUNG FU FOR KIDS	D1880
LOGIC OF VIOLENCE	D2351
NORTHERN SHAOLIN SWORD —SAN CAI JIAN, KUN WU JIAN, QI MEN JIAN	D1194
QIGONG FOR HEALING	D2320
QIGONG FOR LONGEVITY	D2092
QIGONG FOR WOMEN	D2566
SABER FUNDAMENTAL TRAINING	D1088
SHAOLIN KUNG FU FUNDAMENTAL TRAINING—COURSES 1 & 2	D0436
SHAOLIN LONG FIST KUNG FU—BASIC SEQUENCES	D661
SHAOLIN LONG FIST KUNG FU—INTERMEDIATE SEQUENCES	D1071
SHAOLIN LONG FIST KUNG FU—ADVANCED SEQUENCES 1	D2061
SHAOLIN LONG FIST KUNG FU—ADVANCED SEQUENCES 2	D2313
SHAOLIN SABER—BASIC SEQUENCES	D0616
SHAOLIN STAFF—BASIC SEQUENCES	D0920
SHAOLIN WHITE CRANE GONG FU BASIC TRAINING—COURSES 1 & 2	D599
SHAOLIN WHITE CRANE GONG FU BASIC TRAINING—COURSES 3 & 4	D0784
SHUAI JIAO—KUNG FU WRESTLING	D1149
SIMPLE QIGONG EXERCISES FOR ARTHRITIS RELIEF	D0890
SIMPLE QIGONG EXERCISES FOR BACK PAIN RELIEF	D0883
SIMPLIFIED TAI CHI CHUAN—24 & 48 POSTURES	D0630
SUNRISE TAI CHI	D0274
SUNSET TAI CHI	D0760
SWORD—FUNDAMENTAL TRAINING	D1095
TAI CHI BALL QIGONG—COURSES 1 & 2	D0517
TAI CHI BALL QIGONG—COURSES 3 & 4	D0777
TAI CHI CHUAN CLASSICAL YANG STYLE	D645
TAI CHI CONNECTIONS	D0444
TAI CHI ENERGY PATTERNS	D0525
TAI CHI FIGHTING SET	D0509
TAI CHI PUSHING HANDS—COURSES 1 & 2	D0495
TAI CHI PUSHING HANDS —COURSES 3 & 4	D0681
TAI CHI SWORD—CLASSICAL YANG STYLE	D0452
TAIJI & SHAOLIN STAFF—FUNDAMENTAL TRAINING	D0906
TAIJI CHIN NA IN-DEPTH	D0463
TAIJI 37 POSTURES MARTIAL APPLICATIONS	D1057
TAIJI SABER CLASSICAL YANG STYLE	D1026
TAIJI WRESTLING	D1064
UNDERSTANDING QIGONG 1—WHAT IS QI? • HUMAN QI CIRCULATORY SYSTEM	D069X
UNDERSTANDING QIGONG 2—KEY POINTS • QIGONG BREATHING	D0418
UNDERSTANDING QIGONG 3—EMBRYONIC BREATHING	D0555
UNDERSTANDING QIGONG 4—FOUR SEASONS QIGONG	D0562
UNDERSTANDING QIGONG 5—SMALL CIRCULATION	D0753
UNDERSTANDING QIGONG 6—MARTIAL QIGONG BREATHING	D0913
WHITE CRANE HARD & SOFT QIGONG	D637
WUDANG KUNG FU—FUNDAMENTAL TRAINING	D1316
WUDANG SWORD	D1903
WUDANG TAIJIQUAN	D1217
XINGYIQUAN	D1200
YANG TAI CHI FOR BEGINNERS	D2306
YMAA 25 YEAR ANNIVERSARY DVD	D0708

more products available from . . .
YMAA Publication Center, Inc. 楊氏東方文化出版中心

1-800-669-8892 • info@ymaa.com • www.ymaa.com